D0814889

Clinical Calculations

WITH APPLICATIONS TO GENERAL AND SPECIALTY AREAS

W. B. SAUNDERS COMPANY
Harcourt Brace Jovanovich, Inc.

West Washington Square
Philadelphia, PA 19105

Editor: Michael Brown
Developmental Editor: Frances T. Mues
Designer: Karen O'Keefe
Production Manager: Peter Faber
Manuscript Editor: RoseMarie Klimowicz
Illustration Coordinator: Peg Shaw

Notice: The authors and publisher of this book have made every effort to ensure that the dosages of drugs are correct with the standards accepted at the time of publication. The reader is advised to consult the instruction insert of each drug before administering to ascertain any change in drug dosage or method of administration.

Library of Congress Cataloging-in-Publication Data

Kee, Joyce LeFever.
  Clinical calculations.

  Bibliography: p.
  Includes index.
    1. Pharmaceutical arithmetic.   I. Marshall, Sally M.
II. Title.   [DNLM: Drugs—administration & dosage.
QV 748 K26c]
RS57.K44   1988   615'.14   87-32218
ISBN 0-7216-2073-6

Clinical Calculations   ISBN   0-7216-2073-6

Last digit is the print number: 9   8   7   6   5   4   3   2   1

DEDICATIONS

To My MOTHER
and
To My Son DREW

Sally Marshall

To My Grandchildren
CHRISTOPHER, BRENDA, and JESSICA

Joyce Kee

To
OUR NURSING COLLEAGUES

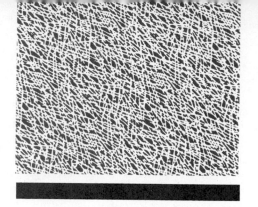

Preface

This text arose from a learning gap that we saw between education and practice. We felt a bridge was needed for the student in understanding the wide range of clinical calculations used in practice. The clinical calculations presented in the specialty areas reflect concepts of drug and fluid administration in a variety of clinical situations.

This clinical calculation book has three major components: systems, conversion, and methods for drug calculation; calculations for administration of oral, injectable, and intravenous drugs; and calculations for clinical specialty areas. The book is useful for nurses in all levels of nursing education who are learning for the first time how to calculate dosage problems, and for beginning practitioners in specialty areas of pediatrics, critical care, labor and delivery, and community. It also can be used in nursing refresher courses, inservice programs, hospital units, home health care, and other places of nursing practice.

The book is divided into four parts. Part I is the basic math review, written concisely for nursing students to review Roman numerals, fractions, decimals, percentage, and ratio and proportion. A post–math review test follows. The math test can be taken first, and if the student has a score of 80% or higher, the basic review section can be omitted. Part II covers metric, apothecary, and household systems used in drug calculations; conversion of units; and methods of calculation. Part III covers calculating drug and fluid dosages for oral, injectable, and intravenous administrations. Clinical drug calculations used in specialty areas are found in Part IV. This part includes pediatrics, critical care for adults and children, labor and delivery, and community. There are five appendices: temperature conversion, conversion table, abbreviations, guidelines for administration of medications, and nomograms.

Each chapter has a content list, objectives, introduction, and numerous practice problems. The practice problems relate to clinical drug problems that are currently used in clinical settings. Illustrations of tablets, capsules, medicine cup, syringes, and drug labels are shown throughout the chapters.

Calculators may be used in solving dosage problems. Many institutions have calculators available. It is suggested that the nurse work the problem without a calculator and then check the answer with a calculator.

We wish to extend our sincere appreciation to the following persons who reviewed chapters of the manuscript and offered helpful suggestions: Dr. Evelyn Hayes, Chairperson of the Department of Nursing Science; Sandra Dunnington, Assistant Professor; Dr. Carolyn Freed, Assistant Professor; Janet Arenson, Obstetric Instructor; Susan Noyes, Obstetric/Pediatric Instructor; Margaret Dada, Pediatric Instructor; Mary Gallagher, Pediatric/Community Instructor; Phyllis Lindvig, Pediatric/Obstetric Instructor—all from the College of Nursing, University of Delaware; Laura Manchester, Inservice Education Instructor at the Medical Center of Delaware; Janis Smith, Pediatric Critical Care Clinical Instructor, University of Pennsylvania; Nancy Murray, Pediatric Nurse Practitioner; Joy Biancosino, Unit Instructor in Labor and Delivery at the Medical Center of Delaware; Theresa Johnston, Unit Instructor in Pediatrics; and Deborah A. Szurgot, Chemist.

Thirty senior nursing students from the College of Nursing, University of Delaware, gave invaluable suggestions and comments: Cheryl Alfes, Eileen Banack, Debbie Belz, Cindy Brown, Kate Burkman, Paula Cammarota, Robin Davis, Christine Demers, Carol Eastham, Lori Goldstein, Elizabeth Grupp, Maureen Harding, Carolyn Hess, Megan Jensen, Lisa Johnson, Crescence Kilcoyne, Carol Lanning, Beverly Laughon, Colleen O'Connor, Allison Parent, Donna Parosky, Mary Piascinski, Linda Porter, Colleen Shaffer, Kim Smida, Linda Smith, Linnea Smith, Heather Spreen, Sally Vanderhey, and Peggy Zurkowski.

Our sincere thanks are extended to the pharmaceutical companies and manufacturers of syringes for their uses of labels and IV syringe/needle displays: Eli Lilly and Co.; Bristol Laboratories, Division of Bristol-Myers Co.; Burroughs Wellcome Co.; Merck, Sharp and Dohme; Mead Johnson Co.; Parke-Davis and Co.; Baxter/Travenol Laboratories; Burron Medical Inc.; and Wyeth Laboratories (Tubex syringe).

We wish to extend our appreciation and love to our husbands, Edward D. Kee and Robert F. Marshall, for their support and suggestions.

Joyce L. Kee
Sally M. Marshall

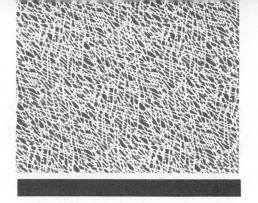

Brief Contents

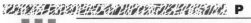 **P   A   R   T**

III CALCULATIONS FOR ORAL, INJECTABLE, AND INTRAVENOUS DRUGS 63

 P   A   R   T

IV CALCULATIONS FOR SPECIALTY AREAS 125

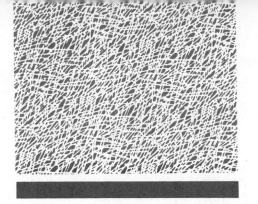

Contents

P   A   R   T

III   CALCULATIONS FOR ORAL, INJECTABLE, AND INTRAVENOUS DRUGS   63

PART

IV CALCULATIONS FOR SPECIALTY AREAS   125

Chapter 7
PEDIATRICS   127

Chapter 8
CRITICAL CARE   141

Chapter 9
PEDIATRIC CRITICAL CARE   173

Chapter 10
LABOR AND DELIVERY   183

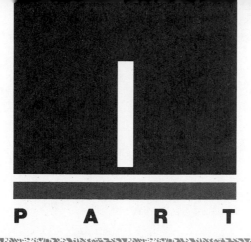

PART

Basic Math Review

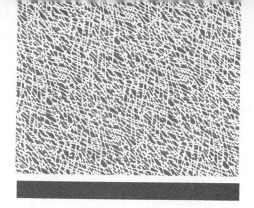

NUMBER SYSTEMS
    Arabic System
    Roman System
    Conversion of Systems

FRACTIONS
    Proper, Improper, and Mixed Fractions
    Multiplying Fractions
    Dividing Fractions
    Decimal Fractions

DECIMALS
    Multiplying Decimals
    Dividing Decimals

RATIO AND PROPORTION

PERCENTAGE

POST-MATH TEST

Objectives

- Convert Roman numerals to Arabic numbers.
- Multiply and divide fractions and decimals.
- Solve ratio and proportion problems.
- Change percentage to decimals, fractions, and ratio and proportion.
- Demonstrate an understanding of Roman numerals, fractions, decimals, ratio and proportion, and percentage by passing the math test.

The basic math review assists nurses in converting Roman and Arabic numerals, multiplying and dividing fractions and decimals, and solving ratio and proportion and percentage problems. Nurses need to master the basic math skills in order to solve drug problems used in the administration of medication.

A math test found on page 14 follows the basic math review. The test may be taken first, and if a score of 80% or greater is achieved, the math review or Part I can be omitted. If the test score is less than 80%, the nurse should do the basic math review section. Some may choose to start with Part I and then take the test.

NUMBER SYSTEMS

Two systems of numbers currently used are Arabic and Roman. Both systems are used in drug administration.

Arabic System

The Arabic system is expressed in numbers 0, 1, 2, 3, 4, 5, 6, 7, 8, 9. These may be written as a whole number or with fractions and decimals. This system is commonly used today.

Roman System

Numbers used in the Roman system are designated by selected capital letters, i.e., I, V, X. Roman letters may be changed to Arabic numbers.

Conversion of Systems

Roman Number	Arabic Number
I	1
V	5
X	10
L	50
C	100

The apothecary system of measurement uses Roman numerals when writing drug dosages. The Roman numerals are written in lower case letters, i.e., i, v, x, xii. The lower case letters may have a line on top of the letters, i.e., $\bar{i}$, $\bar{v}$, $\bar{x}$, $\overline{xii}$.

Roman numerals may appear together, such as xv and ix. To read the multiple Roman numerals, addition and subtraction are used.

METHOD A	If the *first* Roman numeral is *greater* than the following numeral(s), then **ADD**.

EXAMPLES

$$\overline{viii} = 5 + 3 = 8$$
$$\overline{xv} = 10 + 5 = 15$$

METHOD B	If the *first* Roman numeral is *less* than the following numeral(s), then **SUBTRACT**. Subtract the first numeral from the second (smaller from the larger).

EXAMPLES

$$\overline{iv} = 5 - 1 = 4$$
$$\overline{ix} = 10 - 1 = 9$$

Some Roman numerals require both addition and subtraction to obtain the value. Read from left to right.

EXAMPLES

$$\overline{xix} = 10 + 9 \ (10 - 1) = 19$$
$$\overline{xxxiv} = 30 \ (10 + 10 + 10) + 4 \ (5 - 1) = 34$$

Practice Problems

1. $\overline{xvi}$

_____

2. $\overline{xii}$

_____

3. $\overline{xxiv}$

_____

4. $\overline{xxxix}$

_____

5. XLV

_____

6. XC

_____

ANSWERS

1. $10 + 5 + 1 = 16$
2. $10 + 2 = 12$
3. $20 \ (10 + 10) + 4 \ (5 - 1) = 24$
4. $30 \ (10 + 10 + 10) + 9 \ (10 - 1) = 39$
5. $40 \ (50 - 10) + 5 = 45$
6. $100 - 10 = 90$

FRACTIONS

Fractions are expressed as part(s) of a whole or part(s) of a unit. A fraction is composed of two basic numbers: a *numerator* (the top number) and a *denominator* (the bottom number). The denominator indicates the total number of parts.

EXAMPLE

Fraction: $\underline{3}$ numerator (3 of 4 parts)
        4 denominator (4 of 4 parts or 4 total parts)

The value of a fraction depends mainly on the denominator. When the denominator increases, such as $\frac{1}{10}$ to $\frac{1}{20}$, the value of the fraction decreases because it takes more parts to make a whole.

EXAMPLE

Which fraction has the greatest value, $\frac{1}{4}$ or $\frac{1}{6}$? The denominators are 4 and 6.

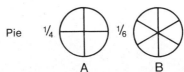

The largest value would be $\frac{1}{4}$ because 4 parts make the whole, whereas for $\frac{1}{6}$ it takes 6 parts to make a whole. Therefore, $\frac{1}{6}$ has the smaller value.

Proper, Improper, and Mixed Fractions

In a *proper fraction* (simple fraction), the numerator is less than the denominator, i.e., $\frac{1}{2}$, $\frac{2}{3}$, $\frac{3}{4}$, $\frac{2}{6}$. When possible, the fraction should be reduced to its lowest term, i.e., $\frac{2}{6} = \frac{1}{3}$ (2 goes into 2 and 6).

In an *improper fraction*, the numerator is greater than the denominator, i.e., $\frac{4}{2}$, $\frac{8}{5}$, $\frac{14}{4}$. Reduce improper fractions to whole numbers or mixed numbers, i.e., $\frac{4}{2} = 2$ ($\frac{4}{2}$ means the same as $4 \div 2$); $\frac{8}{5} = 1\frac{3}{5}$ ($8 \div 5$, 5 goes into 8 one time with 3 left over or $\frac{3}{5}$); and $\frac{14}{4} = 3\frac{2}{4} = 3\frac{1}{2}$ ($14 \div 4$, 4 goes into 14 three times with 2 left over or $\frac{2}{4}$, reduced to $\frac{1}{2}$).

A *mixed number* is a whole number and a fraction, i.e., $1\frac{3}{5}$, $3\frac{1}{2}$. Mixed numbers can be changed to improper fractions by multiplying the denominator by the whole number, then adding the numerator ($1\frac{3}{5} = \frac{8}{5}$).

The apothecary system uses fractions with drug dosage. Fractions may be added, subtracted, multiplied, or divided. Multiplying fractions and dividing fractions are the two common methods used in solving dosage problems.

Multiplying Fractions

In multiplying fractions, multiply the numerator and then the denominator. Reduce the fraction, if possible, to lowest terms.

EXAMPLES

1. $\dfrac{1}{3} \times \dfrac{3}{5} = \dfrac{\overset{1}{\cancel{3}}}{\underset{5}{\cancel{15}}} = \dfrac{1}{5}$

Answer is $\frac{3}{15}$ reduced to $\frac{1}{5}$. In reducing numbers, the number that goes into 3 and 15 is 3. Therefore, 3 goes into 3 one time and 3 goes into 15 five times.

2. $\dfrac{1}{3} \times 6 = \dfrac{6}{3} = 2$

A whole number is considered the numerator over one ($\frac{6}{1}$). Six is divided by 3 ($6 \div 3$); 3 goes into 6 two times.

Dividing Fractions

In dividing fractions, invert the *second fraction* or divisor and then multiply.

EXAMPLES

1. $\dfrac{3}{4} \div \dfrac{3}{8}$ (divisor) $= \dfrac{\overset{1}{\cancel{3}}}{\underset{1}{\cancel{4}}} \times \dfrac{\overset{2}{\cancel{8}}}{\underset{1}{\cancel{3}}} = \dfrac{2}{1} = 2$

When dividing, invert the divisor $\frac{3}{8}$ to $\frac{8}{3}$ and multiply. In reducing to lowest terms, 3 goes into both 3s one time, and 4 goes into 4 and 8 one time and two times.

2. $\dfrac{1}{6} \div \dfrac{4}{18} = \dfrac{1}{\cancel{6}_{1}} \times \dfrac{\cancel{18}^{3}}{4} = \dfrac{3}{4}$

Six and 18 are reduced or cancelled to 1 and 3.

Decimal Fractions

Fractions may be changed to decimals. Divide the numerator by the denominator, i.e., $\frac{3}{4} = 4\overline{)3.00}\,^{0.75}$. Therefore, $\frac{3}{4}$ is the same as 0.75.

Practice Problems

1. Which has the greatest value, $\frac{1}{50}$ or $\frac{1}{100}$?

_____

2. Reduce improper fractions to whole or mixed numbers.

    a. $\frac{12}{4} =$ **c.** $\frac{22}{3} =$

_____   _____

    b. $\frac{20}{5} =$ **d.** $\frac{32}{6} =$

_____   _____

3. Multiply fractions.

    a. $\frac{2}{3} \times \frac{1}{8} =$ **b.** $2\frac{2}{5} \times 3\frac{3}{4} =$

                                      $\frac{12}{5} \times \frac{15}{4} =$

_____   _____

4. Divide fractions.

    a. $\frac{2}{3} \div 6 =$ **b.** $\frac{1}{4} \div \frac{7}{8} =$

_____   _____

    c. $3\frac{2}{3} \div 5\frac{5}{6} =$ **d.** $9\frac{3}{5} \div 4 =$

        $\frac{11}{3} \div \frac{35}{6} =$ $\frac{48}{5} \div \frac{4}{1} =$

_____   _____

5. Change fraction to a decimal.

    a. $\frac{1}{4} =$ **b.** $\frac{1}{10} =$ **c.** $\frac{2}{5} =$

_____   _____   _____

ANSWERS

1. $\frac{1}{50}$ has the greatest value; there are 50 parts in a whole and not 100 parts.

2. a. 3   **c.** $7\frac{1}{3}$

   b. 4   **d.** $5\frac{2}{6}$ or $5\frac{1}{3}$

3. a. $\frac{2}{24} = \frac{1}{12}$ **b.** $\frac{12}{5} \times \frac{15}{4} = 9$

4. a. $\frac{2}{3} \div 6 =$ **b.** $\frac{1}{4} \div \frac{7}{8} =$

   $\frac{2}{3} \times \frac{1}{6} = \frac{1}{9}$ $\frac{1}{4} \times \frac{8}{7} = \frac{2}{7}$

   c. $1\frac{1}{3} \div 3\frac{5}{6} =$ **d.** $48\frac{4}{5} \div \frac{4}{1} =$

   $1\frac{1}{3} \times \frac{6}{35} = \frac{22}{35}$ $48\frac{4}{5} \times \frac{1}{4} = 12\frac{2}{5} = 2\frac{2}{5}$

5. a. $\frac{1}{4} = \quad \begin{array}{r} 0.25 \\ 4\,\overline{)1.00} \end{array}$ **b.** $\frac{1}{10} = \quad \begin{array}{r} 0.10 \\ 10\,\overline{)1.00} \end{array}$

   c. $\frac{2}{5} = \quad \begin{array}{r} 0.40 \\ 5\,\overline{)2.00} \end{array}$

DECIMALS

Decimals are referred to as (1) whole numbers (numbers to the left of decimal point) and (2) decimal fractions (numbers to the right of decimal point). The following number, 2468.8642, is an example of the division of units for a whole number with a decimal fraction.

Whole Numbers					Decimal Fractions			
2 Thousands	4 Hundreds	6 Tens	8 Units	•	8 Tenths	6 Hundredths	4 Thousandths	2 Ten Thousandths

Decimal fractions are written in tenths, hundredths, thousandths, and ten thousandths. Frequently, decimal fractions are used in drug dosing. The metric system is referred to as the decimal system. After solving decimal problems, decimal fractions are rounded off to tenths. To round off in tenths, if the hundredth column is 5 or greater, the tenth is increased by 1, i.e., 0.67 or 0.7 (tenths).

Decimal fractions are an integral part of the metric system. Tenths mean 0.1 or $\frac{1}{10}$, hundredths mean 0.01 or $\frac{1}{100}$, and thousandths mean 0.001 or $\frac{1}{1000}$. When a decimal fraction is changed to a fraction, the denominator is based on the number of digits to the right of the decimal point (0.8 is $\frac{8}{10}$, 0.86 is $\frac{86}{100}$).

EXAMPLES

1. 0.5 is $\frac{5}{10}$ or 5 tenths.

2. 0.55 is $\frac{55}{100}$ or 55 hundredths.

3. 0.555 is $\frac{555}{1000}$ or 555 thousandths.

Multiplying Decimals

To multiply decimal numbers, multiply the multiplicand by the multiplier. Count how many numbers (spaces) are to the right of the decimals in the problem. Mark off the number of decimal spaces in the answer (right to left) according to the number of decimal spaces in the problem. Round off in tenths.

EXAMPLE

$$\begin{array}{r} 1.34 \\ 2.3 \\ \hline 402 \\ 2680 \\ \hline 3.082 \end{array}$$

1.34   multiplicand

2.3   multiplier

3.082   or 3.1 (rounded off in tenths)

Answer: 3.1

Since 8 is 5 or greater than 5, the tenth number is increased by 1.

Dividing Decimals

To divide decimal numbers, the decimal point in the divisor is moved to the right to make a whole number. The decimal point in the dividend is also moved to the right according to the number of decimal spaces in the divisor.

EXAMPLE

$$\text{Dividend} \div \text{Divisor}$$

$$2.46 \div 1.2 \text{ or } \frac{2.46}{1.2} =$$

$$\text{divisor } 1.2\overline{)2.4\,60} \text{ dividend} \quad \frac{2.05}{} = 2.1$$

$$\underline{2\,4}$$
$$60$$
$$\underline{60}$$

Practice Problems

1. Multiply $6.8 \times 0.123 =$

_____

2. Divide $69 \div 3.2 =$

_____

3. Divide $6.63 \div 0.23 =$

_____

4. Change the decimals to fractions.

    a. $0.46 =$ **b.** $0.05 =$ **c.** $0.012 =$

    _____   _____   _____

ANSWERS

1. 0.8364 or 0.8

2. 21.56 or 21.6 (6 hundredths is greater than 5, so tenth is increased by one)

3. 28.826 or 28.8 (2 hundredths is *not* 5 or greater than 5, so the 8 tenths is not changed)

4. a. $^{46}/_{100}$ **b.** $^{5}/_{100}$ **c.** $^{12}/_{1000}$

RATIO AND PROPORTION

A *ratio* is the relationship between two numbers and is separated by a colon, i.e., 1:2 (1 is to 2). It is another way of expressing a fraction, i.e., $1:2 = \frac{1}{2}$.

Proportion is the relationship between two ratios separated by a double colon (: :) or equal (=) sign.

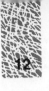

To solve a ratio and proportion problem, the middle numbers (*means*) are multiplied and the end numbers (*extremes*) are multiplied. To solve for the unknown which is X, the X goes first.

EXAMPLES

1. 1 : 2 : : 2 : X (1 is to 2, as 2 is to X)

  X = 4   (1 X is the same as X)

Answer: 4 (1 : 2 : : 2 : 4)

2. 4 : 8 = X : 12

  8 X = 48
  X = $^{48}/_8$ = 6

Answer: 6 (4 : 8 = 6 : 12)

3. The ratio and proportion problem may be set up as a fraction.

Ratio and Proportion	*Fraction*
2 : 3 : : 4 : X	$\frac{2}{3} = \frac{4}{X}$ (cross multiply)
2 X = 12	2 X = 12
X = $^{12}/_2$ = 6	X = 6

Answer: 6.   Remember to cross multiply when the problem is set up as a fraction.

Practice Problems

Solve for X.

1. 2 : 10 : : 5 : X

_____

2. 0.9 : 100 = X : 1000

_____

3. Change ratio and proportion to fraction.

  3 : 5 : : X : 10

_____

4. It is 500 miles from Washington, DC, to Boston, MA. The car is averaging 1 gallon of gas per 22 miles. How many gallons of gasoline will be needed for the trip?

_____

ANSWERS

1. 2 X = 50
      X = 25

2. 100 X = 900
        X = 9

3. $\frac{3}{5} = \frac{X}{10} =$ 5 X = 30
                    X = 6

4. 1 gal: 22 miles : : X gal : 500
        22 X = 500
          X = 22.7 gal
22.7 gallons of gasoline are
needed

PERCENTAGE

Percent (%) means 100. 2% means 2 parts of 100 and 0.9% means 0.9 part (less than 1) of 100. A percent may be expressed as a fraction, a decimal, or a ratio.

EXAMPLE

Percent		Fraction	Decimal	Ratio
60%	=	$\frac{60}{100}$	0.60	60 : 100

NOTE: To change percent to decimal, move the decimal point two places to the left. In the example, the decimal point comes after the whole number 60.

Practice Problems

Change percent to fraction, decimal, and ratio.

	Percent	Fraction	Decimal	Ratio
1.	2%			
2.	½% (0.5%)			
3.	150%			

ANSWERS

	Percent	Fraction	Decimal	Ratio
1.	2	$\frac{2}{100}$	0.02	2 : 100
2.	0.5	$\frac{0.5}{100}$ or $\frac{5}{1000}$	0.005	0.5 : 100 or 5 : 1000
3.	150	$\frac{150}{100}$	1.50	150 : 100

POST-MATH TEST

The math test is composed of five sections: Roman and Arabic numerals, fractions, decimals, ratio and proportion, and percentage. There are 50 questions. Passing score is 40 or more correct answers (80%). Non-passing is 10 incorrect answers.

Roman and Arabic Numerals

Convert Roman numerals to Arabic numerals.

1. $\overline{\text{vii}}$

2. $\overline{\text{xi}}$

3. $\overline{\text{xvi}}$

4. $\overline{\text{xiv}}$

5. xliii or XLIII

Convert Arabic numerals to Roman numerals.

6. 4

7. 18

8. 29

9. 37

10. 62

Fractions

Which fraction has the largest value?

11. $\frac{1}{100}$ or $\frac{1}{150}$?

12. $\frac{1}{3}$ or $\frac{1}{2}$?

Reduce improper fractions to whole or mixed numbers.

13. $\frac{45}{9}$ =

14. $\frac{74}{3}$ =

Change mixed number to improper fraction.

15. $5\frac{2}{3} =$

_____

Change fractions to decimals.

16. $\frac{2}{3} =$ **17.** $\frac{1}{12} =$

_____   _____

Multiply fraction.

18. $\frac{7}{8} \times \frac{4}{6} =$

_____

Divide fractions.

19. $\frac{1}{2} \div \frac{1}{3} =$

_____

20. $6\frac{3}{4} \div 3 =$

_____

Decimals

Round off decimal numbers to tenths.

21. $0.87 =$ **23.** $0.42 =$

_____   _____

22. $2.56 =$

_____

Change decimals to fractions.

24. $0.68 =$ **26.** $0.012 =$

_____   _____

25. $0.9 =$

_____

Multiply decimals.

27. $0.34 \times 0.6 =$

_____

28. $2.123 \times 0.45 =$

_____

Divide decimals.

29. $3.24 \div 0.3 =$

_____

30. $69.4 \div 0.23 =$

_____

Ratio and Proportion

Change ratio to fraction.

31. $3 : 4 =$ **33.** $65 : 90 =$

_____   _____

32. $1 : 175 =$

_____

Solve ratio and proportion problems.

34. $2 : 3 : : 8 : X$

_____

35. $0.5 : 20 : : X : 100$

_____

36. $3 : 100 = X : 1000$

_____

37. $5 : 25 = 10 : X$

_____

Change ratio and proportion to fraction and solve.

38. $1 : 2 : : 4 : X$

_____

39. $5 : 50 : : X : 300$

_____

40. $0.9 : 10 = X : 100$

_____

Percentage

Change percent to fraction.

41. 3%   **42.** 27%   **43.** 1.2%

Change percent to decimals.

44. 8%   **45.** 15%   **46.** 0.9%   **47.** 3.5%

Change percent to ratio.

48. 35%   **49.** 12.5%   **50.** 4%

ANSWERS

Roman and Arabic Numerals

1. 7   **3.** 16   **5.** 43   **7.** $\overline{\text{xviii}}$ **9.** $\overline{\text{xxxvii}}$

2. 11   **4.** 14   **6.** $\overline{\text{iv}}$ **8.** $\overline{\text{xxix}}$ **10.** LXII

Fractions

11. ¹⁄₁₀₀   **13.** 5   **15.** ¹⁷⁄₃   **17.** 0.08   **19.** ½ × ³⁄₁ = ³⁄₂ = 1½

12. ½   **14.** 24⅔   **16.** 0.66 or 0.7   **18.** ²⁸⁄₄₈ or ⁷⁄₁₂

20. $\dfrac{\overset{9}{\cancel{27}}}{4} \times \dfrac{1}{\underset{1}{\cancel{3}}} = \dfrac{9}{4} = 2\dfrac{1}{4}$

Decimals

21. 0.9   **23.** 0.4   **25.** ⁹⁄₁₀   **27.** 0.204   **29.** 10.8

22. 2.6   **24.** ⁶⁸⁄₁₀₀   **26.** ¹²⁄₁₀₀₀   **28.** 0.95535 or 0.96 or 1.0   **30.** 301.739 or 301.7

Ratio and Proportion

31. ¾   **34.** 12   **37.** 50   **39.** $\dfrac{\overset{1}{\cancel{5}}}{\underset{10}{\cancel{50}}} = \dfrac{X}{300}$

32. ¹⁄₁₇₅   **35.** 2.5   **38.** ½ = ⁴⁄ₓ (cross multiply)

33. ⁶⁵⁄₉₀   **36.** 30   X = 8   10 X = 300

                                                                              X = 30

                                                                  40. ⁰·⁹⁄₁₀ = ˣ⁄₁₀₀

                                                                              10 X = 90

                                                                              X = 9

Percentage

41. ³⁄₁₀₀   **46.** 0.009

42. ²⁷⁄₁₀₀   **47.** 0.035

43. ¹²⁄₁₀₀₀   **48.** 35 : 100

44. 0.08   **49.** 12.5 : 100

45. 0.15   **50.** 4 : 100

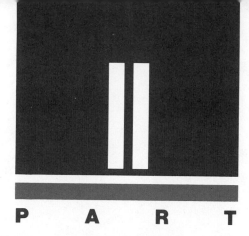

PART II

Systems, Conversion, and Methods of Drug Calculation

METRIC SYSTEM

Conversion Within the Metric System

APOTHECARY SYSTEM

Conversion Within the Apothecary System

HOUSEHOLD SYSTEM

Conversion Within the Household System

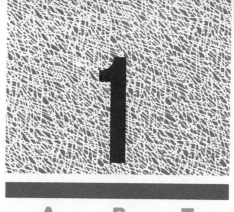

Systems Used for Drug Administration

Objectives

- Recognize the system of measurement accepted worldwide and the system of measurement used in home settings.
- List the basic units and subunits of weight, volume, and length of the metric system.
- Explain the rules for changing grams to milligrams and milliliters to liters.
- Give abbreviations for the frequently used metric units and subunits.
- List the basic units in the apothecary system for weight and volume.
- Give the abbreviations for the apothecary and household units of measurement.
- List the basic units of measurement in the household system for volume.
- Convert units of measurement within the metric system, within the apothecary system, and within the household system.

The three systems used for measuring drugs and solutions are the metric, apothecary, and household. The metric system, developed in 1799 in France, is the chosen system for measurements in the majority of the European countries. The metric system, referred to as the decimal system, is based on 10. Since the enactment of the Metric Conversion Act of 1975, the United States is moving toward the use of this system. The intention of the act is to adopt the International Metric System worldwide by the year 1990.

The apothecary system dates back to the Middle Ages and was the system of weights and measurements used in England since the seventeenth century. This system is referred to as the fractional system since anything less than one is expressed in fractions. In the United States, the apothecary system is rapidly being phased out and is being replaced with the metric system.

Standard household measurements are used primarily in home settings. With the trend toward home care, conversions to household measurements may gain importance.

METRIC SYSTEM

The metric system is a decimal system based on multiples of 10 and fractions of 10. There are three basic units of measurements. The basic units are:

Gram (g, gm, G, Gm)   unit for weight

Liter (l, L)   unit for volume or capacity

Meter (m, M)   unit for linear measurement or length

Prefixes are used with the basic units to describe if the units are larger or smaller than the basic unit. The prefixes indicate the size of the unit in multiples of 10. The prefixes for basic units are:

Prefix for Larger Unit		Prefix for Smaller Unit	
Kilo	1000 (one thousand)	Deci	0.1 (one-tenth)
Hecto	100 (one hundred)	Centi	0.01 (one-hundredth)
Deka	10 (ten)	Milli	0.001 (one-thousandth)
		Micro	0.000001 (one-millionth)
		Nano	0.000000001 (one-billionth)

Abbreviations of metric units that are frequently written in drug orders are listed in Table 1–1. Small letters for abbreviations are usually used rather than capital letters.

TABLE 1–1 Metric Units and Abbreviations

	Names	Abbreviations
Weight	Kilogram	kg, Kg
	Gram	g, gm, G, Gm
	Milligram	mg, mgm
	Microgram	mcg, μg
	Nanogram	ng
Volume	Kiloliter	kl, Kl
	Liter	l, L
	Deciliter	dl
	Milliliter	ml
Length	Kilometer	km, Km
	Meter	m, M
	Centimeter	cm
	Millimeter	mm

The basic units of metric measurements are summarized in Table 1–2. Note that the larger units are 1000, 100, and 10 and the smaller units are 0.1, 0.01, 0.001, 0.000001, and 0.000000001. A basic unit can change size by multiplying or dividing by units of 10. The metric units of weight, volume, and length are given in Table 1–2. Meanings of the prefixes are stated with weights.

TABLE 1–2 Units of Measurement in the Metric System and Their Prefixes

Weight per Grams	Meaning
1 Kilogram (kg) = 1000 grams	one thousand
1 Hectogram (hg) = 100 grams	one hundred
1 Dekagram (dag) = 10 grams	ten
1 Gram (g) = 1 gram	one
1 Decigram (dg) = 0.1 gram ($\frac{1}{10}$)	one-tenth
1 Centigram (cg) = 0.01 gram ($\frac{1}{100}$)	one-hundredth
1 Milligram (mg) = 0.001 gram ($\frac{1}{1000}$)	one-thousandth
1 Microgram (mcg) = 0.000001 gram ($\frac{1}{1,000,000}$)	one-millionth
1 Nanogram (ng) = 0.000000001 gram ($\frac{1}{1,000,000,000}$)	one-billionth

Volume per Liter	Length per Meter
1 Kiloliter (kl) = 1000 liters	1 Kilometer (km) = 1000 meters
1 Hectoliter (hl) = 100 liters	1 Hectometer (hm) = 100 meters
1 Dekaliter (dal) = 10 liters	1 Dekameter (dam) = 10 meters
1 Liter (1, L) = 1 liter	1 Meter (m) = 1 meter
1 Deciliter (dl) = 0.1 liter	1 Decimeter (dm) = 0.1 meter
1 Centiliter (cl) = 0.01 liter	1 Centimeter (cm) = 0.01 meter
1 Milliliter (ml) = 0.001 liter	1 Millimeter (mm) = 0.001 meter

Conversion Within the Metric System

Drug administration often requires conversion within the metric system to prepare the correct dosage. Two basic methods are given for changing larger to smaller units and smaller to larger units.

> **METHOD A**
>
> To change from a **larger** unit to a **smaller** unit, *multiply by 10 for each unit decreased or move the decimal point one space to the right* for each unit changed.
>
> IT DOES *NOT* APPLY TO MICRO AND NANO UNITS.

When changing three units from larger to smaller, such as gram to milligram (a change of three units), multiply 10 three times (or by 1000) or move the decimal point three spaces to the right, e.g., 1 g × 1000 = 1000 mg *or* 1 g = 1.000 mg.

When changing two units, such as kilogram to dekagram (a change of two units from larger to smaller), multiply 10 twice (or by 100) or move the decimal point two spaces to the right, e.g., 2 kg × 100 = 200 dag or 2 kg = 2.00 dag (200 dag).

When changing one unit, such as liter to deciliter (a change of one unit from larger to smaller), multiply by 10 or move the decimal point one space to the right, e.g., 1 L × 10 = 10 dl *or* 1 L = 1.0 dl (10 dl).

Micro unit is one-thousandth of a milli unit and nano unit is one-thousandth of a micro unit. Unit change of micro and nano to its nearest unit is 1000 instead of 10. When changing milli unit to micro units, multiply 1000 or move the decimal point three spaces to the right. The same is true when changing micro unit to nano units.

EXAMPLES

Problem 1:   Change 3 meters to millimeters (a change of three units).

3 meters = 30 decimeters = 300 centimeters = 3000 millimeters

3 × 10   × 10   × 10   = 3000 millimeters

Problem 2:   Change 2 grams to milligrams.

2 g × 1000 = 2000 mg

or

2 g = 2.000 mg (2000 mg)

Problem 3:   Change 10 milligrams to micrograms.

$$10 \text{ mg} \times 1000 = 10{,}000 \text{ mcg } (\mu g)$$

    or

$$10 \text{ mg} = 10.\underset{\curvearrowright}{000} \text{ mcg } (10{,}000 \text{ mcg})$$

Problem 4:   Change 4 liters to milliliters.

$$4 \text{ L} \times 1000 = 4000 \text{ ml}$$

    or

$$4 \text{ L} = 4.\underset{\curvearrowright}{000} \text{ ml } (4{,}000 \text{ ml})$$

Problem 5:   Change 2 kilometers to hectometers.

$$2 \text{ km} \times 10 = 20 \text{ hm}$$

    or

$$2 \text{ km} = 2.\underset{\curvearrowright}{0} \text{ hm } (20 \text{ hm})$$

METHOD B	To change from a **smaller** unit to a **larger** unit, *divide* by 10 for each unit increased *or* move the decimal point *one space to the left* for each unit changed.

When changing three units from smaller to larger, divide by 1000 or move the decimal point three spaces to the left, e.g., liter to kiloliter, 20 L ÷ 1000 = 0.02 kl *or* 20 L = $\underset{\curvearrowright}{020}$. kl (0.02 kl).

When changing two units from smaller to larger, divide by 100 or move the decimal point two spaces to the left, e.g., centimeter to meter, 400 cm ÷ 100 = 4 m *or* 400 cm = 4 $\underset{\curvearrowright}{00}$. m (4 m).

When changing one unit from smaller to larger, divide by 10 or move the decimal point one space to the left, e.g., decigram to gram, 150 dg ÷ 10 = 15 g *or* 150 dg = 15 $\underset{\curvearrowright}{0}$. g (15 g).

EXAMPLES

Problem 1:   Change 8 grams to kilograms.

$$8 \text{ g} \div 1000 = 0.008 \text{ kg}$$

    or

$$8 \text{ g} = \underset{\curvearrowright}{008}. \text{ kg } (0.008 \text{ kg})$$

Problem 2:   Change 1500 milligrams to decigrams.

$$1500 \text{ mg} \div 100 = 15 \text{ dg}$$

or

$$1500 \text{ mg} = 15 \underset{\frown}{00}. \text{ dg (15 dg)}$$

Problem 3:   Change 750 micrograms to milligrams.

$$750 \text{ mcg} \div 1000 = 0.75 \text{ mg}$$

or

$$750 \text{ mcg} = \underset{\frown}{750}. \text{ mg (0.75 mg)}$$

Problem 4:   Change 2400 milliliters to liters.

$$2400 \text{ ml} \div 1000 = 2.4 \text{ L}$$

or

$$2400 \text{ ml} = 2 \underset{\frown}{400}. \text{ L (2.4 L)}$$

Problem 5:   Change 5.5 liters to dekaliters.

$$5.5 \text{ L} \div 10 = 0.55 \text{ dal}$$

or

$$5.5 \text{ L} = \underset{\frown}{5}.5 \text{ dal (0.55 dal)}$$

Practice Problems

1. Conversion from larger units to smaller units: *multiply* by 10 for each unit changed (multiply by 10, 100, 1000) or move the decimal point one space to the *right* for each unit changed (move one, two, or three spaces), Method A.

1.1 7.5 grams to milligrams

_____

1.2 10 milligrams to micrograms

_____

1.3 35 kilograms to grams

_____

1.4 2.5 liters to milliliters

_____

1.5 1.25 liters to milliliters

_____

1.6 20 centiliters to milliliters

_____

1.7 18 decigrams to milligrams

_____

1.8 0.5 kilograms to grams

_____

2. Conversion from smaller units to larger units: *divide* by 10 for each
unit changed (divide by 10, 100, 1000) or move the decimal point one
space to the *left* for each unit changed (move one, two, or three
spaces), Method B.

2.1 500 milligrams to grams

_____

2.2 7500 micrograms to milligrams

_____

2.3 250 grams to kilograms

_____

2.4 4000 milliliters to liters

_____

2.5 325 milligrams to grams

_____

2.6 100 milliliters to deciliters

_____

2.7 2800 milliliters to liters

_____

2.8 75 millimeters to centimeters

_____

ANSWERS

1.1 7.5 g to mg
 7.5 g $\times$ 1000 = 7500 mg
   or
 7.500 mg (7500 mg)

1.2 10,000 mcg

1.3 35,000 g

1.4 2500 ml

1.5 1250 ml

1.6 200 ml

1.7 1800 mg

1.8 500 g

2.1 500 mg to g
 500 $\div$ 1000 = 0.5 g
   or
 500 mg = 500. g (0.5 g)

2.2 7.5 mg

2.3 0.25 kg

2.4 4 L

2.5 0.325 g

2.6 1 dl

2.7 2.8 L

2.8 7.5 cm

TABLE 1–3   Abbreviations and Units of Measurement in the
Apothecary System

Abbreviations			
Weight		**Liquid Volume**	
grain	gr	quart	qt
ounce	oz	pint	pt
dram	dr	fluid ounce	fl oz, fl ℥
		fluid dram	fl dr, fl ℨ
		minim	♏

Basic Equivalent Units			
Weight		**Liquid Volume**	
Larger units	*Smaller units*	*Larger units*	*Smaller units*
1 ounce	= 480 grains	1 quart	= 2 pints
1 ounce	= 8 drams	1 pint	= 16 fluid ounces
1 dram	= 60 grains	1 fluid ounce	= 8 fluid drams
		1 fluid dram	= 60 minims
		1 minim	= 1 drop (gtt)

Note: Constant values are the numbers of the smaller equivalent units.

APOTHECARY SYSTEM

The basic unit of weight in the apothecary system is the grain (gr), and the basic unit of fluid volume is the minim (m); these are the smaller units in the apothecary system. Larger units of measurements for weight and fluid volume are dram (dr or ℨ) and ounce (oz or ℥). In the apothecary system, Roman numerals are written in lower case letters, e.g., gr x, to express numbers. Table 1–3 gives the equivalents of units of weight (grain, dram, ounce) and units of liquid volume (minim, fluid dram, fluid ounce). Since dram and ounce are larger units of weight, it is unlikely that a nurse would administer these units in dry weight. However, do not be surprised to find in clinical practice that dram and ounce are referred to as units of liquid volume, since these measurements are infrequently used as dry weights. The word fluid in front of dram and ounce is dropped. In this text the proper names for units of dry weight and units of liquid volume will be used.

At the present time the apothecary system is being phased out, and in the near future all measurements will be in the metric system. Since there are physicians who still write medication orders using apothecary units, and probably will be for the next several decades, nurses need to know and to interpret the apothecary system.

Conversion Within the Apothecary System

It is often necessary to change units within the apothecary system. The method applied when changing larger units to smaller units is:

METHOD C	To change a **larger** unit to a **smaller** unit, *multiply* the constant value found in Table 1–3 by the number(s) of the larger unit.

NOTE: The constant values are the basic equivalent numbers of the smaller units given in Table 1–3. You might want to memorize these equivalents or refer to the table as needed.

EXAMPLES

Problem 1: 2 drams (dr) = _____ grains (gr).

$$1 \text{ dr} = 60 \text{ gr (60 is the constant value)}$$

$$2 \times 60 = 120 \text{ grains}$$

Problem 2: ½ ounce (oz or ℥) = _____ grains (gr).

$$1 \text{ oz} = 480 \text{ gr (480 is the constant value)}$$

$$½ \times 480 = 240 \text{ grains}$$

Problem 3: 4 fluid drams (fl ℈) = _____ minims (m).

$$1 \text{ fl dr} = 60 \text{ minims (60 is the constant value)}$$

$$4 \times 60 = 240 \text{ minims}$$

Problem 4: 3 fluid ounces (fl ℥) = _____ fluid drams (fl ℈).

$$1 \text{ fl oz} = 8 \text{ fl dr (8 is the constant value)}$$

$$3 \times 8 = 24 \text{ fluid drams}$$

The method applied when changing smaller units to larger units is:

METHOD D	To change a **smaller** unit to a **larger** unit, *divide* the constant value found in Table 1–3 into the number(s) of the smaller unit.

EXAMPLES

Problem 1: 30 grains (gr) = _____ dram (dr or ℈).

$$60 \text{ gr} = 1 \text{ dr (60 is the constant value)}$$

$$30 \div 60 = ½ \text{ dram}$$

Problem 2: 20 drams (dr) = _____ ounces (oz or **3**).

$$8 \text{ dr} = 1 \text{ oz } (8 \text{ is the constant value})$$

$$20 \div 8 = 2\frac{1}{2} \text{ ounces}$$

Problem 3: 180 minims (m) = _____ fluid drams (fl **3**).

$$60 \text{ minims} = 1 \text{ fl dr } (60 \text{ is the constant value})$$

$$180 \div 60 = 3 \text{ fluid drams}$$

Problem 4: 2 fluid drams (fl **3**) = _____ fluid ounce (fl **3**).

$$8 \text{ fl dr} = 1 \text{ fl oz } (8 \text{ is the constant value})$$

$$2 \div 8 = \frac{1}{4} \text{ fluid ounce}$$

Practice Problems

1. Give the abbreviations for:

1.1 grain = _____

1.2 dram = _____

1.3 fluid dram = _____

1.4 minim = _____

1.5 drop = _____

1.6 fluid ounce = _____

1.7 pint = _____

1.8 quart = _____

2. Give the equivalent using Method C, changing larger units to smaller units.

2.1 3 v = _____ gr

2.2 fl **3** v = _____ fl 3

2.3 qt iii = _____ pt

2.4 pt ii = _____ fl 3

2.5 fl **3** iiss = _____ m

3. Give the equivalent using Method D, changing smaller units to larger units.

3.1 gr 240 = _____ dr or 3

3.2 **3** xvi = _____ oz or **3**

3.3 fl **3** xxiv = _____ fl 3

3.4 m xxx = _____ fl 3

3.5 m xv = _____ gtts

ANSWERS

Abbreviations	*Equivalents*	*Equivalents*
1.1 grain = gr	**2.1** ℥ v = _____ gr 5 × 60 = 300 gr	**3.1** gr 240 = _____ dr 240 ÷ 60 = 4 ℥
1.2 dram = dr or ℥	**2.2** 40 fl ℥	**3.2** 2 oz or ℥
1.3 fluid dram = fl ℥ , fl dr	**2.3** 6 pt	**3.3** 3 fl ℥
1.4 minim = m	**2.4** 32 fl ℥	**3.4** ½ fl ℥
1.5 drop = gtt	**2.5** 150 m	**3.5** 15 gtts
1.6 fluid ounce = fl ℥ , fl oz		
1.7 pint = pt		
1.8 quart = qt		

HOUSEHOLD SYSTEM

The use of household measurements is on the increase because more patients/clients are being cared for in the home. The household system of measurement is not as accurate as the metric system owing to a lack of standardization of spoons, cups, and glasses. A teaspoon (t) is considered 5 ml although it could be anywhere from 4 to 6 ml. Three household teaspoons equal one tablespoon (T); however, according to the metric and apothecary systems, four teaspoons equal one calibrated tablespoon. A drop size can vary with the size of the lumen of the dropper. Basically, a drop and a minim are considered equal. Again, household measurements must be considered as approximate measures. Some of the household units are the same as the apothecary units, for there is a blend of these two systems.

The community health nurse may have to use and teach the household units of measurements to patients/clients.

Table 1–4 gives the commonly used units of measurement in the household system. You might want to memorize the equivalents in Table 1–4 or refer to the table as needed.

TABLE 1–4   Units of Measurement in the Household System   _____

1 drop (gtt)	= 1 minim (m)
1 teaspoon (t)	= 60 drops (gtts)
1 tablespoon (T)	= 3 teaspoons (t)
1 ounce (oz)	= 2 tablespoons (T)
1 coffee cup (c)	= 6 ounces (oz)
1 medium size glass	= 8 ounces (oz)
1 measuring cup	= 8 ounces (oz)

Note: Constant values are the numbers of the smaller equivalent units.

Conversion Within the Household System

For changing larger units to smaller units and smaller units to larger units within the household system, the same methods that applied to the apothecary system can be used.

METHOD E	To change a **larger** unit to a **smaller** unit, *multiply* the constant value found in Table 1–4 by the number(s) of the larger unit.

NOTE: The constant values are the basic equivalent numbers of the smaller units in Table 1–4.

EXAMPLES

Problem 1: 2 medium size glasses = _____ ounces (oz).

1 medium glass = 8 fl oz (8 is the constant value)

$2 \times 8 = 16$ oz

Problem 2: 3 tablespoons (T) = _____ teaspoons (t).

1 T = 3 t (3 is the constant value)

$3 \times 3 = 9$ t

Problem 3: 5 ounces (oz or ℥) = _____ tablespoons (T).

1 oz = 2 T (2 is the constant value)

$5 \times 2 = 10$ T

Problem 4: 2 teaspoons (t) = _____ drops (gtts).

1 t = 60 gtts (60 is the constant value)

$2 \times 60 = 120$ gtts

METHOD F	To change a **smaller** unit to a **larger** unit, *divide* the constant value found in Table 1–4 into the number(s) of the smaller unit.

EXAMPLES

Problem 1: 120 drops (gtts) = _____ teaspoons (t).

1 t = 60 gtts (60 is the constant value)

$120 \div 60 = 2$ t

Problem 2:   6 teaspoons (t) = _____ tablespoons (T).

$$1 \text{ T} = 3 \text{ t } (3 \text{ is the constant value})$$

$$6 \div 3 = 2 \text{ T}$$

Problem 3:   18 ounces (oz) = _____ cups (c).

$$1 \text{ c} = 6 \text{ oz } (6 \text{ is the constant value})$$

$$18 \div 6 = 3 \text{ c}$$

Problem 4:   4 tablespoons (T) = _____ ounces (oz).

$$1 \text{ oz} = 2 \text{ T } (2 \text{ is the constant value})$$

$$4 \div 2 = 2 \text{ oz}$$

Practice Problems

1. Give the equivalents using Method E, changing larger units to smaller units.

1.1 2 glasses = _____ oz

1.2 3 ounces = _____ T

1.3 4 tablespoons = _____ t

1.4 1½ cups = _____ oz

1.5 ½ teaspoon = _____ gtts

2. Give the equivalents using Method F, changing smaller units to larger units.

2.1 9 teaspoons = _____ T

2.2 6 tablespoons = _____ oz

2.3 90 drops = _____ t

2.4 12 ounces = _____ c

2.5 24 ounces = _____ medium size glasses

ANSWERS

1.1 2 glasses = _____ oz
$2 \times 8 = 16 \text{ oz}$

1.2 6 T

1.3 12 t

1.4 9 oz

1.5 30 gtts

2.1 9 teaspoons = _____ T
$9 \div 3 = 3 \text{ T}$

2.2 3 oz

2.3 1½ t

2.4 2 c

2.5 3 glasses

SUMMARY PRACTICE PROBLEMS

1. Metric System

    1.1 30 mg = _____ mcg

    1.2 3 g = _____ mg

    1.3 6 L = _____ ml

    1.4 1.5 kg = _____ g

    1.5 10,000 mcg = _____ mg

    1.6 500 mg = _____ g

    1.7 2500 ml = _____ L

    1.8 125 g = _____ kg

    1.9 120 mm = _____ cm

    1.10 5 m = _____ cm

2. Apothecary System

    2.1 90 gr = _____ dr

    2.2 fl ℥ iv = _____ fl ʒ

    2.3 fl ʒ iiss = _____ fl ℥

    2.4 m xxx = _____ fl ℥

    2.5 8 pt = _____ qt

    2.6 fl ʒ ii = _____ m

3. Household System

    3.1 12 t = _____ T

    3.2 5 glasses = _____ oz

    3.3 3 T = _____ t

    3.4 2 c = _____ oz

    3.5 4 oz = _____ T

    3.6 12 gtts = _____ m

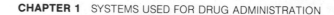

ANSWERS

1.1 30,000 mcg
1.2 3000 mg
1.3 6000 ml
1.4 1500 g
1.5 10 mg

1.6 0.5 g
1.7 2.5 L
1.8 0.125 kg
1.9 12 cm
1.10 500 cm

2.1 1.5 ʒ
2.2 ½ or ss fl ʒ
2.3 20 fl ʒ
2.4 ½ or ss fl ʒ
2.5 4 qt
2.6 120 m̅

3.1 4 T
3.2 40 oz
3.3 9 t
3.4 12 oz
3.5 8 T
3.6 12 m̅

UNITS AND MILLIEQUIVALENTS
METRIC, APOTHECARY, AND HOUSEHOLD EQUIVALENTS

Conversion in Metric and Apothecary Systems by Weight

Conversion in Metric, Apothecary, and Household Systems by Volume

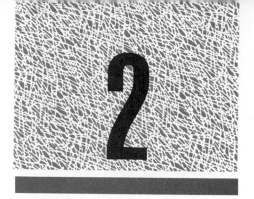

Conversion Within the Metric, Apothecary, and Household Systems

Objectives

- State rules for converting drug dosage by weight between the apothecary and metric systems.
- Convert grams/milligrams to grains, and grains to grams/milligrams.
- Convert drug dosage by weight from one system to another system using the ratio method.
- State rules for converting drug dosage by volume between the metric, apothecary, and household systems.
- Convert liters/milliliters to ounces and pints, and milliliters to drams, tablespoons, and teaspoons.

Drug doses are usually ordered in metric units (grams, milligrams, liters, and milliliters). Although the apothecary system is phasing out, there are some physicians who still order drug doses by apothecary units. To calculate a drug dose, the same unit of measurement must be used. Therefore, the nurse must know the metric and apothecary equivalents either by memorizing the equivalent table or by using methods for converting from one system to the other. Once the conversion to one system is made, the dosage problem can be solved. Some authorities state it is easier to convert to the unit used on the container (bottle). If the physician ordered phenobarbital gr ½ and the bottle is labeled 30 mg, then the conversion would be from grains to milligrams.

Metric and apothecary equivalents are approximations, such as 1 gram equals 15.432 grains. When values are unequal, they should be rounded off to the nearest whole number (1 gram = 15 grains).

Dosage conversion tables are available in many institutions; however, at times when you need a conversion table, one might not be found. Again, nurses should either memorize metric and apothecary equivalents or be able to convert from one system to the other by using calculation methods.

UNITS AND MILLIEQUIVALENTS

Units and milliequivalents are two methods used to indicate the strength or potency of certain drugs. When all drugs are developed, their strength is based on either chemical assay or biological assay. Chemical assay denotes strength by weight, e.g., milligrams or grains. Biological assays are used for drugs when the chemical composition is difficult to determine. Biological assays assess potency by the effect one *unit* of the drug may have on a laboratory animal. Units mainly measure the potency of hormones, vitamins, anticoagulants, and some antibiotics. Drugs that were once standardized by units and later synthesized to their chemical composition may still retain units as an indication of potency, e.g., insulin.

Milliequivalents measure the strength of an ion concentration. Ions are given primarily for electrolyte replacement. They are measured in milliequivalents, mEq, which is ¹/₁₀₀₀ of the equivalent weight of an ion. Potassium chloride, KCl, is a common electrolyte replacement and is ordered in mEq.

Units and milliequivalents cannot be directly converted to the metric, apothecary, or household system.

METRIC, APOTHECARY, AND HOUSEHOLD EQUIVALENTS

Knowing how to convert drug doses between the systems of measurement is essential in the clinical setting. In discharge teaching for individuals receiving liquid medication, converting metric to household measurement may be important.

Table 2–1 gives the metric and apothecary equivalents by weight, and the metric, apothecary, and household equivalents by volume.

TABLE 2–1 Approximate Metric, Apothecary, Household Equivalents

	Metric System	Apothecary System	Household System
Weight	30 grams	1 ounce	
	15 grams	4 drams	
	*1 g; 1000 mg	15 (16) gr	
	0.5 g; 500 mg	7 ½ gr	
	0.3 g; 300 mg	5 gr	
	0.1 g; 100 mg	1 ½ gr	
	*0.06 g; 60 (65) mg	1 gr	
	0.03 g; 30 (32) mg	½ gr	
	0.01 g; 10 mg	⅙ gr	
	0.6 mg	$\frac{1}{100}$ gr	
	0.4 mg	$\frac{1}{150}$ gr	
	0.3 mg	$\frac{1}{200}$ gr	
Volume	1 L; 1000 ml (cc)	1 qt; 32 fl oz (fl ʒ)	1 qt
	0.5 L; 500 ml	1 pt; 16 fl oz	1 pt
	0.24 L; 240 ml	8 oz	1 glass
	0.18 L; 180 ml	6 oz	1 cup
	*30 ml	1 oz or 8 dr (fl ʒ)	2 T or 6 t
	15 ml	½ oz or 4 dr	1 T (tbsp)
	4–5 ml		1 t (tsp)
	4 ml	1 dr or 60 minims (m)	1 t (tsp)
	1 ml	15 (16) m	15–16 gtts
Other	1 kg; 1000 grams	2.2 lb	

*Equivalents commonly used for computing conversion problems by ratio.
Note: ½ may be written as ss.

Remember, conversion from one system to the other is an approximate equivalent. Either memorize the table or use the methods that follow in the text for system conversion.

Conversion in Metric and Apothecary Systems by Weight

METHOD A   **Grams and grains:** 1 g = 15 gr

> **a.** To convert grams to grains, *multiply* the number of grams by 15, the constant value.
> **b.** To convert grains to grams, *divide* the number of grains by 15, the constant value.

EXAMPLES

Problem 1:   Change 2 grams to grains.

$$2 \times 15 = 30 \text{ gr (grains)}$$

Problem 2:   Change 60 grains to grams.

$$60 \div 15 = 4 \text{ g (grams)}$$

METHOD B   **Grains and milligrams:** 1 gr = 60 mg

> **a.** To convert grains to milligrams, *multiply* the number of grains by 60, the constant value.
> **b.** To convert milligrams to grains, *divide* the number of milligrams by 60, the constant value.

EXAMPLES

Problem 1:   Change 3 grains to milligrams.

$$3 \times 60 = 180 \text{ mg (milligrams)}$$

Problem 2:   Change 300 milligrams to grains.

> *NOTE:*   325 milligrams may be ordered instead of 300. Round off to the whole number. One grain is equivalent to 60 or 64 or 65

milligrams. In this situation you may want to divide by 65 instead of rounding off to the whole number.

$$300 \div 60 = 5 \text{ gr (grains)}$$

or

$$325 \div 65 = 5 \text{ gr}$$

or

$$325 \div 60 = 5.43 \text{ gr or 5 gr (0.43 is less than 0.5)}$$

If it is difficult for you to recall these methods, then use the ratio and proportion to convert from one system to the other.

You must memorize:

> 1 gram = 1000 milligrams
> 1 gram = 15 grains
> 1 grain = 60 milligrams

Ratio and proportion   Multiply the means (numbers that are closer to each other) by the extremes (numbers that are farthest from each other). You are solving for X, so it goes first.

EXAMPLES

Problem 1:   Convert 2.5 grams to grains.

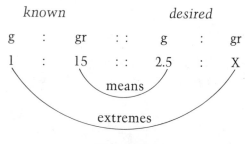

$$X = 37.5 \text{ gr}$$

Problem 2:   Convert 10 grains to milligrams.

$$
\begin{array}{ccccccc}
\text{\textit{known}} & & & & \text{\textit{desired}} & & \\
\text{gr} & : & \text{mg} & : : & \text{gr} & : & \text{mg} \\
1 & : & 60 \text{ (65)} & : : & 10 & : & \text{X}
\end{array}
$$

$$X = 600 \text{ mg or 650 mg}$$

> *NOTE:* Since conversion gives approximate values, the answer could be 600 mg or 650 mg. If the problem uses 1 gr = 60 mg, the answer is 600 mg. However, the bottle may be labeled 10 gr = 650 mg. Both 600 mg and 650 mg would be correct.

Practice Problems

Method A

1. 10 g = _____ gr

2. 0.5 g = _____ gr

3. 0.1 g = _____ gr

4. 0.03 g = _____ gr

5. 3 gr = _____ g

6. 1 ½ gr = _____ g

Method B

1. 4 gr = _____ mg

2. 1 ½ gr = _____ mg

3. 7 ½ gr = _____ mg

4. ½ gr = _____ mg

5. 150 mg = _____ gr

6. 30 mg = _____ gr

Ratio and proportion

1. 2.5 g = _____ mg

2. 0.5 g = _____ gr

3. 1 gr = _____ g

4. ¼ gr = _____ mg

ANSWERS

Method A

1. 10 × 15 = 150 gr
2. 0.5 × 15 = 7.5 or 7 ½ gr
3. 0.1 × 15 = 1.5 or 1 ½ gr

4. 0.03 × 15 = 0.45 or 0.5 gr
5. 3 ÷ 15 = 0.2 g
6. 1.5 ÷ 15 = 0.1 g

Method B

1. 4 × 60 = 240 mg
2. 1.5 × 60 = 90 (100) mg
3. 7.5 × 60 = 450 mg

4. 0.5 × 60 = 30 mg
5. 150 ÷ 60 = 2.5 or 2 ½ gr
6. 30 ÷ 60 = 0.5 or ½ gr

Ratio and proportion

1. g : mg :: g : mg
  1 : 1000 :: 2.5 : X
   X = 2500 mg

or

Move decimal point three spaces to the right (conversion within the metric system)

$$2.5 \text{ g} = 2.500 \text{ mg}$$

2. g : gr :: g : gr
  1 : 15 :: 0.5 : X
  X = 7.5 or 7 ½ gr

3. g : gr :: g : gr
  1 : 15 :: X : 1
  15 X = 1
  X = 0.06 g

4. gr : mg :: gr : mg
  1 : 60 :: 0.25 : X
  X = 60 × 0.25
  X = 15 mg

Conversion in Metric, Apothecary, and Household Systems by Volume

METHOD C **Liters and ounces:** 1 L = 32 oz

a. To convert liters and quarts to ounces, *multiply* the number of liters by 32, the constant value.

b. To convert ounces to liters or quarts, *divide* the number of ounces by 32, the constant value.

EXAMPLES

Problem 1: Change 3 liters to ounces.

$$3 \text{ L} \times 32 = 96 \text{ oz or f } \textbf{3} \text{ (ounces)}$$

Problem 2: Change 64 ounces to liters.

$$64 \text{ oz} \div 32 = 2 \text{ L (liters)}$$

METHOD D **Ounces and milliliters:** 1 oz = 30 ml

a. To convert ounces to milliliters, *multiply* the number of ounces by 30, the constant value.

b. To convert milliliters to ounces, *divide* the number of milliliters by 30, the constant value.

EXAMPLES

Problem 1:   Change 5 ounces to milliliters.

$$5 \text{ oz} \times 30 = 150 \text{ ml (milliliters) or cc}$$

Problem 2:   Change 120 milliliters to ounces.

$$120 \text{ ml} \div 30 = 4 \text{ oz or f } 3 \text{ (ounces)}$$

METHOD E   **Milliliters and drops:** 1 ml = 15 drops (gtts) or
15 minims

> **a.** To convert milliliters to minims or drops, *multiply* the number of milliliters by 15, the constant value.
> **b.** To convert minims and drops to milliliters, *divide* the number of minims or drops by 15, the constant value.

EXAMPLES

Problem 1:   Change 4 milliliters to minims and drops.

$$4 \text{ ml} \times 15 = 60 \text{ minims or 60 drops}$$

Problem 2:   Change 10 drops (gtts) to milliliters.

$$10 \text{ m or gtts} \div 15 = \tfrac{2}{3} \text{ ml or 0.667 ml or 0.7 ml}$$

If it is difficult for you to recall these methods, then use the ratio and proportion to convert from one system to the other.
You must memorize:

$$30 \text{ ml} = 1 \text{ oz} = 8 \text{ dr} = 2T = 6t$$

These are equivalent values.

Ratio and proportion: Again the ratio method is useful when converting smaller units within the three systems.

EXAMPLES

Problem 1:   Change 20 ml to teaspoons.

known			*desired*	
ml	:	t	::	ml	:	t
30	:	6	::	20	:	X

$$30 \text{ X} = 120$$
$$X = 4 \text{ t (teaspoons)}$$

Problem 2:   Change 15 ml to tablespoons.

known   *desired*

ml   :   T   ::   ml   :   T

30   :   2   ::   15   :   X

$$30 \text{ X} = 30$$
$$\text{X} = 1 \text{ T (tablespoon)}$$

Problem 3:   Change 5 oz to tablespoons.

known   *desired*

oz   :   T   ::   oz   :   T

1   :   2   ::   5   :   X

$$\text{X} = 10 \text{ T (tablespoons)}$$

SUMMARY PRACTICE PROBLEMS

Before computing dosage problems, one system of measurement must be selected. If a medication is ordered in one system and the drug label is in another system, then conversion to one of the systems is necessary. As previously stated, it may be easier to convert to the system used on the drug label.

There are three methods of conversion for the three systems: (1) memorization of a conversion table, (2) conversion methods, and (3) ratio method. You need to convert not only within three systems, but also within the same system if units are not the same, e.g., grams and milligrams. Again, units of measurement *must* be the same to solve problems.

Remember: *Multiply* when converting from larger to smaller units, and *divide* when converting from smaller to larger units.

Weight: Metric and Apothecary Conversion

A. To convert grams to grains, _____ the number of grams by _____, and to convert grains to grams, _____ the number of grains by _____.

    1. 2 g = _____ gr   **4.** 0.02 g = _____ gr

    2. 7 ½ gr (gr v̄iīss) = _____ g   **5.** 150 gr = _____ g

    3. 3 gr = _____ g   **6.** 0.06 g = _____ gr

B. To convert grains to milligrams, _____ the number of grains by _____, and to convert milligrams to grains, _____ the number of milligrams by _____.

1. 3 gr (gr iii) = _____ mg   **4.** 5 gr = _____ mg

2. 10 mg = _____ gr   **5.** 7½ gr = _____ mg

3. ¼ gr = _____ mg   **6.** 0.4 mg = _____ gr

C. Ratio

Remember: 1 g or 1000 mg = 15 gr; 60 (65) mg = 1 gr

1. Change 5 g to gr

_____

2. Change 120 mg to gr

_____

Volume:
Metric, Apothecary, and
Household Conversion

D. To convert liters and quarts to ounces, _____ the number of liters by _____, and to convert ounces to liters and quarts, _____ the number of ounces by

_____.

1. 3 L = _____ oz (fl ʒ)   **4.** ½ L = _____ oz

2. 1½ qt = _____ oz   **5.** 8 oz = _____ L or qt

3. 64 oz (fl ʒ) = _____ qt   **6.** 24 oz = _____ qt

E. To convert ounces to milliliters, _____ the number of ounces by _____, and to convert milliliters to ounces, _____ the number of milliliters by _____.

1. 1½ oz = _____ ml   **4.** 75 ml = _____ oz (fl ʒ)

2. 15 ml = _____ oz (fl ʒ)   **5.** 3 oz (fl ʒ) = _____ ml

3. 60 ml = _____ oz   **6.** 8 oz = _____ ml

F. To convert milliliters to minims or drops, _____ the

number of milliliters by _____, and to convert minims

or drops to milliliters, _____ the number of minims or

drops by _____.

1. 15 ml = _____ m or gtts   **4.** 4 ml = _____ m or gtts

2. 10 gtts = _____ ml   **5.** 30 m or gtts = _____ ml

3. 18 m or gtts = _____ ml   **6.** ½ ml = _____ gtts

G. Ratio

Remember: 30 ml = 1 oz = 8 dr = 2 T = 6 t

1. Change 16 oz (fl **з**) to L or qt

_____

2. Change 1½ oz to T

_____

3. Change 1 T to t

_____

4. Change 20 ml to t (teaspoons)

_____

5. Change 2½ oz to ml

_____

6. Change 4 oz to ml

_____

ANSWERS

A. multiply, 15, divide, 15

    1. 2 g × 15 = 30 gr   **4.** 0.02 g × 15 = 0.3 or ⅓ gr

    2. 7.5 gr ÷ 15 = ½ or 0.5 g   **5.** 150 gr ÷ 15 = 10 g

    3. 3 gr ÷ 15 = 0.2 g   **6.** 0.06 g × 15 = 0.9 or 1 gr

                                                 (round off to 1)

B. multiply, 60, divide, 60

    1. 3 gr × 60 = 180 mg   **4.** 5 gr × 60 = 300 mg

    2. 10 mg ÷ 60 = ¹⁰⁄₆₀ = ⅙ gr   **5.** 7.5 gr × 60 = 450 mg

    3. 0.25 gr × 60 = 15 mg   **6.** 0.4 mg ÷ 60 = ⁴⁄₆₀₀ = ¹⁄₁₅₀ gr

C. Ratio and Proportion

1.   *known*   *desired*

g	:	gr	: :	g	:	gr
1	:	15	: :	5	:	X

$$X = 75 \text{ gr}$$

2.
gr	:	mg	: :	gr	:	mg
1	:	60	: :	X	:	120

$$60 \, X = 120$$
$$X = 2 \text{ gr}$$

or

mg	:	gr	: :	mg	:	gr
60	:	1	: :	120	:	X

$$60 \, X = 120$$
$$X = 2 \text{ gr}$$

D. multiply, 32, divide, 32

     1. $3 \text{ L} \times 32 = 96 \text{ oz}$

     2. $1.5 \text{ qt} \times 32 = 48 \text{ oz}$

     3. $64 \text{ oz} \div 32 = 2 \text{ qt}$

     4. $0.5 \text{ L} \times 32 = 16 \text{ oz}$

     5. $8 \text{ oz} \div 32 = {}^{8}\!/_{32} = \frac{1}{4} \text{ L}$

     6. $24 \text{ oz} \div 32 = {}^{24}\!/_{32} = \frac{3}{4} \text{ qt}$

E. multiply, 30, divide, 30

     1. $1\frac{1}{2} \text{ oz} \times 30 = 45 \text{ ml}$

     2. $15 \text{ ml} \div 30 = {}^{15}\!/_{30} = \frac{1}{2} \text{ oz}$

     3. $60 \text{ ml} \div 30 = 2 \text{ oz}$

     4. $75 \text{ ml} \div 30 = 2\frac{1}{2} \text{ oz}$

     5. $3 \text{ oz} \times 30 = 90 \text{ ml}$

     6. $8 \text{ oz} \times 30 = 240 \text{ ml}$

F. multiply, 15, divide, 15

     1. $15 \text{ ml} \times 15 = 225 \text{ m or gtts}$

     2. $10 \text{ gtts} \div 15 = {}^{10}\!/_{15} = \frac{2}{3} \text{ ml}$

     3. $18 \text{ m or gtts} \div 15 = 1\frac{1}{5} \text{ ml}$

     4. $4 \text{ ml} \times 15 = 60 \text{ m or gtts}$

     5. $30 \text{ m or gtts} \div 15 = 2 \text{ ml}$

     6. $\frac{1}{2} \text{ ml} \times 15 = 7.5 \text{ gtts}$

G. Ratio and Proportion

known   *desired*

1. L   :   oz   : :   L   :   oz
    1   :   32   : :   X   :   16

$$32\,X = 16$$
$$X = \tfrac{1}{2}\ L$$

2. oz   :   T   : :   oz   :   T
    1   :   2   : :   1½   :   X

$$X = 3\ T$$

3. T   :   t   : :   T   :   t
    2   :   6   : :   1   :   X

$$2\,X = 6$$
$$X = 3\ t$$

4. ml   :   t   : :   ml   :   t
  30   :   6   : :   20   :   X

$$30\,X = 120$$
$$X = 4\ t$$

5. oz   :   ml   : :   oz   :   ml
    1   :   30   : :   2½   :   X

$$X = 75\ ml$$

6. oz   :   ml   : :   oz   :   ml
    1   :   30   : :   4   :   X

$$X = 120\ ml$$

BASIC FORMULA
RATIO AND PROPORTION
FRACTIONAL EQUATION
BODY WEIGHT
BODY SURFACE AREA

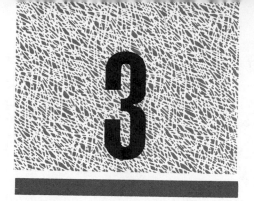

C H A P T E R

Methods of Calculation

Objectives

- Determine the amount of drug needed for a specified period of time.
- Select a dosage formula such as basic formula, ratio and proportion, or fraction equation for calculating drug dosage problems.
- Convert units of measurement to the same system and unit of measurement prior to calculating drug dosage.
- Calculate the dosage/amount of tablets, capsules, and liquid volume (oral or parenteral) needed for administering the prescribed drug.
- Calculate drug dosage needed according to body weight and body surface area.

Before calculating drug dosage, units of measurement must be converted to one system. If the drug is ordered in milligrams and comes in grains, then grains are converted to milligrams or milligrams are converted to grains.

Three methods for calculating drug dosages are the basic formula, ratio and proportion, and fractional equation. *The nurse should choose one of the first three methods for calculating dosages* and stay with the selected method when solving dosage problems. For drugs that require individualized dosing, body weight and body surface area are used. When body weight and body surface area are necessary, one of the first three methods for calculation will be needed.

At some institutions, the nurse orders enough medication doses for a designated period of time. If the order would require 2 tablets, qid (4 times a day) for 5 days, then the number of tablets needed would be 2 tablets × 4 times a day × 5 days = 40 tablets.

METHOD 1: BASIC FORMULA

This formula is frequently used to calculate drug dosages. Since the basic formula is easy to recall, it is a popular one.

$$\frac{D \text{ (desired dose)}}{H \text{ (on hand dose)}} \times V \text{ (vehicle—tablet, liquid)} = \text{Amount to give}$$

D or desired dose: Drug dose ordered by physician.

H or on hand dose: Drug dose on label of container (bottle, vial, ampule).

V or vehicle: Form and amount in which the drug comes (tablet, capsule, liquid).

EXAMPLES

Problem 1: Order: phenytoin/Dilantin 50 mg, p.o., tid.
Drug available: Dilantin 125 mg/5 ml.

   a. No conversion is needed since the units of measurement for the drug ordered and on the label of the bottle are the same.

   b. $\frac{D}{H} \times V = {}^{50}\!/_{125} \times 5 \text{ ml} = {}^{250}\!/_{125} = 2 \text{ ml}$

Answer: Phenytoin/Dilantin 50 mg = 2 ml.

Problem 2: Order: 0.5 g of ampicillin, p.o., bid.
Drug available: ampicillin 250 mg per capsule.

   a. The unit of measurement that is ordered and the unit on the bottle are in the same system but of different units; therefore, conversion of units within the same system must be done first. To convert grams to milligrams, move the decimal point three spaces to the right (see Chapter 1, Metric System).

$$0.5 \text{ g} = .500 \text{ mg} = 500 \text{ mg}$$

b. $\dfrac{D}{H} \times V = {}^{500}/_{250} \times 1$ capsule $= {}^{500}/_{250} = 2$ capsules

Answer: Ampicillin 0.5 g = 2 capsules.

Problem 3:   Order: phenobarbital gr ii, stat.
Drug available: phenobarbital 30 mg per tablet.

a. Before calculating drug dosage, convert to one unit of measurement. To convert grains to milligrams, *multiply* the number of grains by 60 (see Chapter 2, Method B).

$$2 \text{ gr} \times 60 = 120 \text{ mg}$$

b. $\dfrac{D}{H} \times V = {}^{120}/_{30} \times 1 = {}^{120}/_{30} = 4$ tablets

Answer: Phenobarbital gr ii = 4 tablets.

Problem 4:   Order: meperidine/Demerol 35 mg, IM, stat.
Drug available: Demerol in a prefilled syringe labeled 50 mg per 1 ml.

a. Conversion is not needed since both are of the same unit of measurement.

b. $\dfrac{D}{H} \times V = {}^{35}/_{50} \times 1 \text{ ml} = {}^{35}/_{50} = 0.7 \text{ ml}$

Answer: Meperidine/Demerol 35 mg = 0.7 ml.

METHOD 2: RATIO AND PROPORTION

This is the oldest method used for calculating dosage problems.

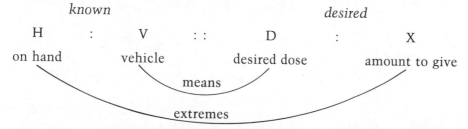

H and V: The left side of the equation are the known quantities, which are dose on hand and vehicle.

D and X: The right side of the equation is the desired dose and the unknown amount to give.

Multiply the means and the extremes. Solve for X.

EXAMPLES

Problem 1:   Order: Keflex 1 g, p.o., bid.
Drug available: Keflex 250 mg per capsule.

    a. Both the dosage of the drug ordered and the dosage on the bottle are in the metric system; however, the units of measurement are different. Conversion is needed. To convert grams to milligrams, move the decimal point three spaces to the right of the gram (see Chapter 1, Metric System).

$$1.0 \text{ g} = 1.000 \text{ mg} = 1000 \text{ mg}$$

    b.

H	:	V	: :	D	:	X
250 mg	:	1 capsule	: :	1000 mg	:	X capsule

$$250 \text{ X} = 1000$$
$$\text{X} = 4 \text{ capsules}$$

Answer: Keflex 1 g = 4 capsules.

NOTE: With ratio and proportion, the ratio on the left, milligrams to capsules, has the same relationship as the ratio on the right, milligrams to capsules; the only difference is values.

Problem 2:   Order: aspirin/ASA gr x, PRN.
Drug available: aspirin 325 mg per tablet.

    a. Convert to one system and unit of measurement. To convert grains to milligrams, *multiply* the number of grains by 60 (65) (see Chapter 2, Method B).

$$10 \text{ gr} \times 60 \ (65) = 600 \text{ or } 650 \text{ mg}$$

or

gr	:	mg	: :	gr	:	mg
1	:	60 (65)	: :	10	:	X

$$\text{X} = 600 \text{ or } 650 \text{ mg}$$

    b.

H	:	V	: :	D	:	X
325	:	1	: :	600 (650)	:	X

$$325 \text{ X} = 600 \ (650)$$
$$\text{X} = 1.8 \text{ tablets or 2 tablets}$$
(round off or use 650 instead of 600)

Answer: Aspirin gr x = 2 tablets.

Problem 3: Order: amoxicillin 75 mg, p.o., qid.
Drug available: amoxicillin 125 mg/5 ml.

a. Conversion is not needed since both are the same units of measurement.

b.

H	:	V	: :	D	:	X
125 mg	:	5 ml	: :	75 mg	:	X ml

$$125 \text{ X} = 375$$
$$\text{X} = 3 \text{ ml}$$

Answer: Amoxicillin 75 mg = 3 ml.

Problem 4: Order: meperidine/Demerol 60 mg, IM, stat.
Drug available: Demerol in a prefilled syringe labeled 100 mg/l ml.

a. Conversion is not needed; same unit of measurement.

b.

H	:	V	: :	D	:	X
100	:	1	: :	60	:	X

$$100 \text{ X} = 60$$
$$\text{X} = 0.6 \text{ ml}$$

Answer: Meperidine/Demerol 60 mg = 0.6 ml.

METHOD 3: FRACTIONAL EQUATION

This method is similar to ratio and proportion, except it is written as a fraction.

$$\frac{H}{V} = \frac{D}{X}$$

H: The dosage on hand or on the container.

V: The vehicle or the form in which the drug comes (tablet, capsule, liquid).

D: The desired dosage.

X: The unknown amount to give.

Cross multiply and solve for X.

EXAMPLES

Problem 1:   Order: Digoxin 0.25 mg, p.o., qd.
Drug available: 0.125 mg per tablet.

a. No unit conversion is needed.

b. $\dfrac{H}{V} = \dfrac{D}{X}$ $\dfrac{0.125 \text{ mg}}{1} = \dfrac{0.25 \text{ mg}}{X}$

$$0.125 \text{ X} = 0.25$$
$$\text{X} = 2 \text{ tablets}$$

Answer: Digoxin 0.25 mg = 2 tablets.

Problem 2:   Order: valproic acid/Depakene 100 mg, p.o., tid.
Drug available: valproic acid/Depakene 250 mg/5 ml suspension.

a. No unit conversion is needed.

b. $\dfrac{H}{V} = \dfrac{D}{X}$ $\dfrac{250}{5} = \dfrac{100}{X} =$

$$250 \text{ X} = 500$$
$$\text{X} = 2 \text{ ml}$$

Answer: Valproic acid/Depakene 100 mg = 2 ml.

Problem 3:   Order: atropine gr $\frac{1}{100}$, IM, stat.
Drug available: atropine in vial, 0.4 mg per 1 ml.

a. Two systems are involved, apothecary (grains) and metric (milligrams). Because the drug preparation is in milligrams, convert grains to milligrams. (See Table 2–1: 0.6 mg = gr $\frac{1}{100}$.)

Also, you could use the ratio method.

gr	:	mg	: :	gr	:	mg
1	:	60	: :	$\frac{1}{100}$	:	X

$$\text{X} = {}^{60}\!/_{100}$$
$$\text{X} = 0.6 \text{ mg}$$

b. $\dfrac{H}{V} = \dfrac{D}{X}$ $\dfrac{0.4}{1} \times \dfrac{0.6}{X} =$

$$0.4 \text{ X} = 0.6$$
$$\text{X} = 1.5 \text{ ml}$$

Answer: Atropine gr $\frac{1}{100}$ = 1.5 ml.

BODY WEIGHT

Body weight allows for the individualizing of the drug dose and is often used for children and patients receiving chemotherapy. The first step is to convert pounds to kilograms (if necessary). The second step is to determine drug dose per body weight by multiplying drug dose × body weight × frequency (day or per day in divided doses). The third step is to choose one of the three methods for drug calculation for the amount of drug to be given.

EXAMPLES

Problem 1:   Order: fluorouracil/5-FU, 12 mg/kg/day intravenously (IV) not to exceed 800 mg/day. The adult weighs 140 pounds.

    a. Convert pounds to kilograms. Divide number of pounds by 2.2. *Remember:* 1 kg = 2.2 lb.

$$140 \div 2.2 = 64 \text{ kg}$$

    b. mg × kg × 1 day =
        12 × 64 × 1   = 768 mg IV per day

Answer: Fluorouracil/5-FU 12 mg/kg/day = 768 mg or 750 to 800 mg.

Problem 2:   Give cefaclor/Ceclor 20 mg/kg/daily in three divided doses. The child weighs 20 pounds.

    a. Convert pounds to kilograms.

$$20 \div 2.2 = 9 \text{ kg}$$

    b. 20 mg × 9 kg × 1 day = 180 mg per day.

$$180 \text{ mg} \div 3 \text{ divided doses} = 60 \text{ mg}$$

    c. The bottle is labeled 125 mg/5 ml.

$$\frac{D}{H} \times V \quad \frac{60}{125} \times 5 = \qquad or \qquad \begin{array}{ccccccc} H & : & V & :: & D & : & X \\ 125 & : & 5 & :: & 60 & : & X \end{array} \qquad or \qquad \frac{125}{5} = \frac{60}{X}$$

$$\frac{300}{125} = 2.4 \text{ ml} \qquad\qquad \begin{array}{rl} 125 \text{ X} &= 300 \\ \text{X} &= 2.4 \text{ ml} \end{array} \qquad\qquad \begin{array}{rl} 125 \text{ X} &= 300 \\ \text{X} &= 2.4 \text{ ml} \end{array}$$

Answer: Cefaclor/Ceclor 20 mg/kg/day = 2.4 ml per dose (3 × a day)

BODY SURFACE AREA OF ADULTS — NOMOGRAM

Height	Body surface area (BSA)	Weight

cm	inch	m²	kg	lb
200	79		150	330
	78	2.80	145	320
195	77	2.70	140	310
	76		135	300
190	75	2.60		290
	74	2.50	130	280
185	73	2.40	125	270
	72		120	260
180	71	2.30	115	250
	70			
175	69	2.20	110	240
	68		105	230
170	67	2.10	100	220
	66			
165	65	2.00	95	210
	64	1.95	90	200
160	63	1.90		190
	62	1.85	85	180
155	61	1.80	80	
	60	1.75		170
150	59	1.70	75	160
	58	1.65		
145	57	1.60	70	150
	56	1.55		
140	55	1.50	65	140
	54	1.45		
135	53	1.40	60	130
	52			
130	51	1.35	55	120
	50	1.30		
125	49	1.25	50	110
	48	1.20		105
120	47	1.15	45	100
	46	1.10		95
115	45		40	90
	44	1.05		85
110	43	1.00		80
	42		35	75
105	41	0.95		
	40	0.90		70
cm 100			kg 30	66 lb
	39 in	0.86 m²		

From: Loebl, S., and Spratto G. *The Nurses' Drug Handbook* 4th ed. New York, John Wiley & Sons, 1986, p. 931. Used by permission. Reproduced from Documenta Geigy Scientific Tables, 8th ed. Courtesy CIBA-GEIGY Limited, Basle, Switzerland, 1981.

BODY SURFACE AREA (BSA)

BSA is considered to be the most accurate way to calculate drug dosage for infants and children, as well as for patients on chemotherapy. The body surface area, square meter (m^2), is determined by the person's height and weight and where they intersect the nomogram scale (see Figure 3–1). To calculate drug dosage by BSA, multiply the drug dose $\times m^2$, e.g., 100 mg $\times$ 1.6 = 160 mg/day.

EXAMPLES

Problem 1:   Order: cyclophosphamide/Cytoxan 100 mg/m² day, p.o. Patient weighs 150 pounds and is 5'8" (68 inches) tall.

    a. 68 inches and 150 pounds intersect the nomogram scale at 1.88 m² (BSA).

    b. 100 mg $\times$ 1.88 = 188 mg/day of Cytoxan.

Answer: Cyclophosphamide/Cytoxan 100 mg/m²/day = 188 mg/day.

Problem 2:   Order: cytarabine/cytosine 200 mg/m²/day IV $\times$ 5 days for patient with myelocytic leukemia. Patient is 64 inches tall and weighs 130 pounds.

    a. 64 inches and 130 pounds intersect the nomogram scale at 1.7 m² (BSA).

    b. 200 mg $\times$ 1.7 = 340 mg IV daily for 5 days of cytarabine.

Answer: Cytarabine/cytosine 200 mg/m²/day = 340 mg/day.

SUMMARY PRACTICE PROBLEMS

Solve the following calculation problems using the formula you have selected. Extra practice problems are available in chapters on orals, injectables, and pediatrics.

1. Order: dexamethasone/Hexadrol 1 mg.
Drug available: dexamethasone/Hexadrol 0.5 mg per tablet.

---

2. Order: sulfisoxazole/Gantrisin 1 g.
Drug available: sulfisoxazole/Gantrisin 250 mg per tablet.

---

3. The physician has ordered erythromycin 500 mg q8h for 7 days. It comes in a 250 mg tablet. How many tablets should you order for 7 days? How many tablets would you give every 8 hours?

---

4. Order: dicloxacillin 125 mg q8h.
   Drug available: dicloxacillin 62.5 mg per 5 ml.

   _____

5. Order: phenobarbital gr 1.
   Drug available: phenobarbital 15 mg per tablet.

   _____

6. Order: cimetidine/Tagamet 0.6 g p.o.
   Drug available: Tagamet 300 mg per tablet.

   _____

7. Order: methylprednisolone/Medrol 75 mg IM.
   Drug available: Medrol 125 mg per 2 ml per ampule.

   _____

8. Order: Keflex gr 7 ½ (gr $\overline{\text{viiss}}$).
   Drug available: Keflex 250 mg per capsule.
   Convert grains to grams and then grams to milligrams.

   _____

9. Order: sulfisoxazole/Gantrisin 50 mg/kg daily in 4 divided doses
   (q6h). The patient weighs 44 pounds.

   _____

10. Order: sulfisoxazole/Gantrisin 2 g/m² daily in 4 divided doses, q6h.
    The patient weighs 110 pounds and is 60 inches tall. See nomogram.

    _____

11. Order: amikacin/Amikin 15 mg/kg/daily in 3 divided doses (q8h) IV.
    Drug is to be diluted in 100 ml of D_5W. The patient weighs 180
    pounds and is 6′ (72 inches).

    _____

12. Order: Adriamycin 60 mg/m² IV per month. Patient weighs 120
    pounds and is 5′2″ (62 inches) tall. See nomogram, Fig. 3–1.

    _____

ANSWERS

1. $\dfrac{D}{H}\dfrac{1}{0.5} \times 1 =$ or   H : V :: D : X   or $\dfrac{0.5}{1} = \dfrac{1}{X}$
                                                      0.5 : 1 :: 1 : X

   $\dfrac{1}{0.5} = 2$ tabs $0.5\,X = 1$ $0.5\,X = 1$
                                      $X = 2$ tabs $X = 2$ tabs

2. 4 tablets.

3. 2 tablets $\times$ 3 doses per day $\times$ 7 days = 42 tablets.
2 tablets every 8 hours.

4. $\dfrac{D}{H} \times V$ $\dfrac{125}{62.5} \times 5 =$ or   H   :   V   ::   D   :   X
                                                                    62.5 :   5   :: 125 :   X

$\quad\quad\dfrac{625}{62.5} = 10$ ml $\quad\quad$ 62.5 X = 625
$\quad\quad\quad\quad\quad\quad\quad\quad\quad\quad\quad$ X = 10 ml

or $\dfrac{62.5}{5} = \dfrac{125}{X}$

$\quad$ 62.5 X = 625
$\quad\quad\quad$ X = 10 ml

5. Change grains to milligrams. Multiply the number of grains by 60.

$\quad\quad\quad$ 1 gr $\times$ 60 = 60 mg (Chapter 2, Method B)

Give 4 tablets.

6. Change grams to milligrams by moving the decimal point at grams, three spaces to the right. Give 2 tablets.

7. $\dfrac{D}{H} \times V$ $\dfrac{75}{125} \times 2 =$ or H   :   V   ::   D   :   X or $\dfrac{125}{2} = \dfrac{75}{X}$
                                                                     125 :   2   :: 75 :   X

$\quad\dfrac{150}{125} = 1.2$ ml $\quad\quad$ 125 X = 150 $\quad\quad\quad$ 125 X = 150
$\quad\quad\quad\quad\quad\quad\quad\quad\quad$ X = 1.2 ml $\quad\quad\quad\quad\quad$ X = 1.2 ml

8. Change gr 7 ½ to grams. Divide the number of grains by 15.

$\quad\quad\quad$ 7.5 $\div$ 15 = 0.5 g (Chapter 2, Method B)

Change grams to milligrams by moving the decimal at the grams three spaces to the right (Chapter 1, Metric System).

$\quad\quad\quad$ 0.5 g = .500 mg = 500 mg

Give 2 capsules.

9. Change 44 pounds to kilograms. 44 $\div$ 2.2 = 20 kg.

$\quad\quad\quad$ 50 mg $\times$ 20 kg $\times$ 1 = 1000 mg of Gantrisin per day

$\quad\quad\quad$ 1000 mg $\div$ 4 times a day (q6h) = 250 mg q6h

10. 60 inches and 110 pounds intersect the nomogram scale at 1.5 m^2.

$\quad\quad\quad$ 2 g $\times$ 1.5 m^2 = 3 g or 3000 mg per day

$\quad\quad\quad$ 3000 mg $\div$ 4 times a day = 750 mg

11. Change 180 pounds to kilograms. $180 \div 2.2 = 81.8$ or 82 kg.

$$15 \text{ mg} \times 82 \text{ kg} \times 1 = 1230 \text{ mg per day}$$

$$1230 \div 3 \text{ times a day (q8h)} = 410 \text{ mg q8h}$$

12. 62 inches and 120 pounds intersect the nomogram scale at 1.6 m^2.

$$60 \text{ mg} \times 1.6 \text{ m}^2 = 96 \text{ mg of Adriamycin}$$

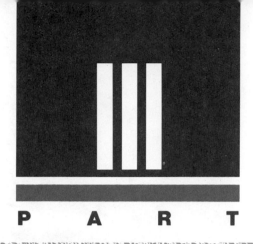

PART

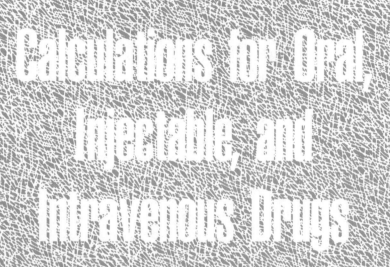

Calculations for Oral, Injectable, and Intravenous Drugs

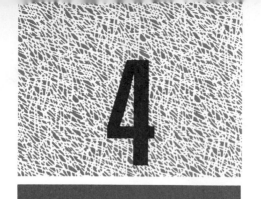

4

C H A P T E R

Oral Preparations with Clinical Applications

Objectives

- State the advantages and disadvantages of administering oral medications.
- Calculate oral dosages from tablets, capsules, and liquids using given formulas.
- Give the rationale for diluting and not diluting oral liquid medications.
- Explain the method for administering sublingual medication.
- Calculate oral medications according to body weight and body surface area.
- Determine the amount of tube feeding solution needed for dilution according to the percentage ordered.

Oral administration of drugs is considered a most convenient and economical method to give medications. Oral drugs are available as tablets, capsules, powders, and liquids. Oral medications are referred to as p.o. (per os, or by mouth) drugs and are absorbed by the gastrointestinal tract, mainly from the small intestine.

There are some disadvantages in administering oral medications, such as: (1) variation in absorption rate due to gastric and intestinal pH and food consumption within the gastrointestinal tract; (2) irritation to the gastric mucosa causing nausea, vomiting, or ulceration, e.g., oral potassium chloride; (3) retention or inactivation of the drug in the body due to partial liver function; (4) destruction of drugs by digestive enzymes; (5) aspiration into the lungs by seriously ill or confused patients; and (6) discoloration of tooth enamel, e.g., SSKI. Oral administration is an effective way to give medications in many instances, and at times it is the route of choice.

TABLETS AND CAPSULES

Most tablets are scored and can be broken in halves (sometimes quarters). Half of a tablet may be indicated when the drug does not come in a lesser strength.

Capsules are gelatin shells containing powder or time pellets. Capsules should remain intact and not be divided in any way. Many drugs that come in capsules also come in liquid form. When a smaller dose is indicated and is not available in tablet or capsule, the liquid form of the drug is used.

Caution:

- A tablet that is NOT scored *should not* be broken.
- Time-released capsules *should not* be crushed and diluted, since the entire medication could be absorbed rapidly.
- Enteric-coated tablets must NOT be crushed, since the medication could irritate the stomach. Enteric-coated tablets are absorbed by the small intestines.
- Tablets/capsules that are irritating to the gastric mucosa should be taken with 6 to 8 ounces of fluid, with meals, or immediately after meals.

Tablets   Scored Tablets   Capsules

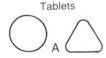 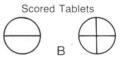 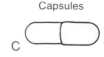

Calculation of Tablets and Capsules

Decide which of the 3 methods of calculation you wish to use and then use that same method for calculating all dosages. In the following examples the basic formula and the ratio and proportion methods will be used.

Basic Formula   *Ratio and Proportion*

$$\frac{D \text{ (desired dose)}}{H \text{ (on hand dose)}} \times V_{\text{(vehicle)}} = \qquad \underset{\text{on hand}}{H} : \underset{\text{vehicle}}{V} :: \underset{\text{desired dose}}{D} : \underset{X}{X}$$

EXAMPLES

Problem 1:   Order: nifedipine/Procardia 20 mg tid.

Drug available: Procardia 10 mg per tablet.

Methods:

$$\frac{D}{H} \times V \qquad\qquad \begin{array}{ccccccc} H & : & V & :: & D & : & X \\ 10 & : & 1 & :: & 20 & : & X \end{array}$$

$$\frac{20}{10} \times 1 = 2 \text{ tablets} \qquad\qquad \begin{array}{l} 10\,X = 20 \\ X = 2 \text{ tablets} \end{array}$$

Answer: Procardia 20 mg = 2 tablets, tid.

Problem 2:   Order: cephalexin/Keflex 0.5 g qid.

Drug available:

Usual Adult Dose— One PULVULE every 6 hours. For more severe infections, dose may be increased, not to exceed 4 g a day. See literature. Each PULVULE contains Cephalexin Monohydrate equivalent to 250 mg Cephalexin.	NDC 0777-0869-02 ℞ 100 PULVULES® No. 402 **KEFLEX®** **CEPHALEXIN CAPSULES, USP** **250 mg** CAUTION—Federal (U.S.A.) law prohibits dispensing without prescription.	Keep Tightly Closed Store at Controlled Room Temperature 59° to 86°F (15° to 30°C) Dispense in a tight container. YD 6040 DPX DISTA PRODUCTS CO. Division of Eli Lilly and Company Indianapolis, IN 46285, U.S.A.

NOTE: Since gram (g) and milligram (mg) are in the metric system, you would change g to mg, or mg to g. Remember in changing g (larger unit) to mg (smaller unit), you move the decimal point three spaces to the *right*. Refer to Chapter 2.

Methods: 0.5 g = .500 mg (Method A)

$$\frac{D}{H} \times V =$$

H : V :: D : X
250 : 1 :: 500 : X

$$\frac{500}{250} \times 1 =$$

250 X = 500
X = 2 tablets

$$\frac{500}{250} = 2 \text{ tablets}$$

Answer: Keflex 0.5 g = 2 tablets.

Problem 3: Order: atropine gr $\frac{1}{150}$, p.o., bid.
Drug available:

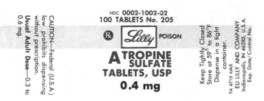

NOTE: Since the atropine bottle is labeled in mg, convert gr to mg. See Table 2-1 or the conversion table in Appendix B. To work out the dosage problem, the system and weight must be the same.

$$\text{gr } \frac{1}{150} = 0.4 \text{ mg}$$

Methods:

$$\frac{D}{H} \times V =$$

H : V :: D : X
0.4 : 1 :: 0.4 : X

$$\frac{0.4}{0.4} \times 1 =$$

0.4 X = 0.4
X = 1 tablet

$$\frac{0.4}{0.4} = 1 \text{ tablet}$$

Answer: Atropine gr $\frac{1}{150}$ = 1 tablet.

Problem 4: Order: aspirin gr x, p.o., stat.
Drug available: aspirin 325 mg per tablet.

NOTE: The dose is ordered in the apothecary system, gr x, and the label on the drug bottle is in the metric system (325 mg). Use Table 2–1 or the conversion table in Appendix B.

$$325 \text{ mg} = \text{gr v (5) and } 650 \text{ mg} = \text{gr x (10)}$$

thods:

$$\frac{D}{H} \times V = \frac{10 \text{ gr}}{5 \text{ gr}} \times 1 = \frac{10}{5} = 2 \text{ tablets}$$

H : V :: D : X
5 : 1 :: 10 : X

or

$$\frac{D}{H} \times V = \frac{650 \text{ mg}}{325 \text{ mg}} \times 1 = \frac{650}{325} = 2 \text{ tablets}$$

5 X = 10
X = 2 tablets

Answer: Aspirin gr x = 2 tablets.

LIQUIDS

Liquid medications come in forms of tincture, elixir, suspension, and syrup. Some liquid medications are irritating to the gastric mucosa and must be well diluted before given, e.g., KCl (potassium chloride). Usually liquid cough medicines are not diluted. Medications in tincture form are always diluted.

tion:

- Concentrated liquid medication that can irritate the gastric mucosa should be diluted in *at least* 4 ounces or more of fluid.
- Liquid medication that can discolor the teeth *should be* well diluted and taken through a drinking straw.

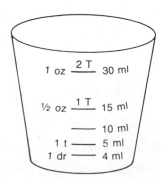

Calculation of Liquid Medication

EXAMPLES

Problem 1:   Order: potassium chloride (KCl) 20 mEq, bid.

Drug available: liquid potassium chloride 10 mEq per 5 ml.

Methods:

$$\frac{D}{H} \times V =$$

$$\frac{20}{10} \times 5 =$$

$$\frac{100}{10} = 10 \text{ ml}$$

H : V :: D : X
10 : 5 :: 20 : X

10 X = 100
X = 10 ml

Answer: Potassium chloride 20 mEq = 10 ml.

Problem 2:   Order: cloxacillin/Tegopen 0.25 g, p.o., tid.

Drug available:

Lot
Exp. date of powder
STORE RECONSTITUTED SOLUTION IN
REFRIGERATOR; discard after 14 days.
KEEP BOTTLE TIGHTLY CLOSED
**Be sure to take each dose prescribed
by your physician.**
NDC 0015-7941-40   7941400RL-04

BRISTOL LABORATORIES
Div. of Bristol-Myers Company, Syracuse, New York 13201
Usual Dosage: Adults—250 mg q. 6h. Children—
50 mg/Kg/day in equally divided doses at 6-hour
intervals.

READ ACCOMPANYING CIRCULAR
To the Pharmacist: Prepare solution at time of dispensing. Add a total of 63 ml water to the bottle.
For ease in preparation, add the water in two portions—shake well after each addition. Bottle then
contains 100 ml of solution; each 5 ml contains
cloxacillin sodium monohydrate equivalent to 125
mg cloxacillin.
© Bristol Laboratories

BRISTOL®   NDC 0015-7941-40
100 ml BOTTLE
LIFT HERE

Tegopen ® CLOXACILLIN
SODIUM FOR ORAL SOLUTION
EQUIVALENT TO

125 mg
per 5 ml CLOXACILLIN
when reconstituted according to directions

CAUTION: Federal law prohibits
dispensing without prescription.

Change g to mg: 0.25 g = 0.250 mg

Methods:

$$\frac{D}{H} \times V =$$

$$\frac{250}{125} \times 5 =$$

$$\frac{1250}{125} = 10 \text{ ml}$$

H : V :: D : X
125 : 5 :: 250 : X

125 X = 1250
X = 10 ml

Answer: Cloxacillin 0.25 g = 10 ml.

Problem 3:   Give SSKI 300 mg q6h diluted in water.

Available: saturated solution of potassium iodide 50 mg/
drop (gtt).

Methods:

$$\frac{D}{H} \times V = \frac{300}{50} \times 1 =$$

$$\frac{300}{50} = 6 \text{ gtts}$$

$$H : V :: D : X$$
$$50 : 1 :: 300 : X$$

$$50 \text{ X} = 300$$
$$X = 6 \text{ gtts}$$

Answer: SSKI 300 mg = 6 gtts (drops).

SUBLINGUAL TABLETS

Few drugs are administered sublingually (tablet placed under the tongue). The sublingual tablets are small and soluble, and are quickly absorbed by numerous capillaries on the underside of the tongue.

tion:

- *Do not* swallow a sublingual tablet, e.g., nitroglycerin (NTG). If the drug is swallowed, the desired immediate action of the drug would be decreased or lost.
- Fluids *should not* be taken until the drug has been dissolved.

Calculation of Sublingual Medication

EXAMPLES

Problem 1: Order: nitroglycerin (NTG) 0.6 mg sublingually.

Drug available:

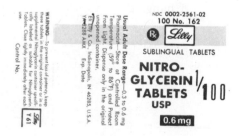

NOTE: The systems and weights must be the same. See Table 2–1 or the conversion table in Appendix B. The label has both systems of measurement.

$$0.6 \text{ mg} = \text{gr } \frac{1}{100}$$

Methods:

$$\frac{D}{H} \times V =$$

$$H : V :: D : X$$

$$\frac{1}{100} : 1 :: \frac{1}{100} : X$$

$$\frac{0.6}{0.6} \times 1 =$$

$$\frac{1}{100} X = \frac{1}{100}$$

$$\frac{0.6}{0.6} = 1 \text{ tablet}$$

$$X = \frac{1}{100} \times \frac{100}{1} = 1 \text{ tablet}$$

Answer: Nitroglycerin/NTG 0.6 mg = 1 tablet.

Problem 2: Order: isosorbide dinitrate (Isordil) 10 mg sublingually.

Drug available: Isordil 5 mg per tablet.

Method:

$$\frac{D}{H} \times V =$$

$$H : V :: D : X$$
$$5 : 1 :: 10 : X$$

$$\frac{10}{5} \times 1 = 2 \text{ tablets}$$

$$5 X = 10$$
$$X = 2 \text{ tablets}$$

Answer: Isordil 10 mg = 2 tablets.

BODY WEIGHT AND BODY SURFACE AREA

The most individualized methods for calculating drug dosage are by body weight and by body surface area. The dose is usually ordered according to the patient's body weight in kilograms or body surface area in square meters (m^2). Usually cancer chemotherapeutic drug dosages are determined by two methods: (1) drug amount × kilograms (mg/kg/day) and (2) body surface area (height and weight intersecting the body surface area on the nomogram). Body surface area is the calculation method frequently selected by pediatricians (see Chapter 7, *Pediatrics*). These methods are considered safe and desirable for selected drug administration and are becoming more widely used. Use the nomogram in Chapter 3 or Appendix E.

Calculation by Body Weight and Body Surface Area

For calculation purposes, 1 kilogram (kg) = 2.2 pounds. Daily doses are usually divided into two to four time periods per day.

ation:

> • Many cancer chemotherapeutic agents are ordered by mg/kg/day. Check patient's weight daily before administering the drug.

EXAMPLES

Problem 1: Order: cyclophosphamide/Cytoxan 2 mg/kg/day, p.o.

Patient weighs 132 pounds.

What is the patient's weight in kg?

How much Cytoxan should be administered?

Method: 132 lb ÷ 2.2 = 60 kg

2 mg × 60 = 120 mg of Cytoxan per day

Answer: Cyclophosphamide/Cytoxan 2 mg/kg/day = 120 mg/day.

Problem 2: Order: mercaptopurine 100 mg/m^2, per day, p.o.

Patient's height is 70 inches and weight is 170 pounds.

How much mercaptopurine should be administered?

Method: The square meters (m^2) is determined according to the nomogram (see Chapter 3, Appendix E). Height and weight intersect on the nomogram at 2.0 m^2.

100 mg × 2.0 = 200 mg of mercaptopurine

Answer: Mercaptopurine 100 mg/m^2 = 200 mg per day.

PERCENTAGE OF SOLUTIONS

Patients may be fed through a nasogastric tube (tube feeding) if they are unable to take nourishment by mouth. Initially the tube feeding may be diluted with water, then gradually increased in strength. Dilutions of tube feeding are ordered in percentage. It is believed that patients tolerate tube feeding better if given gradually in increasing strengths.

Oral medications in liquid, tablet, or capsule forms can be administered through the tube, but should NOT be mixed with the entire tube feeding solution. Mixing medications in a large volume of tube feeding decreases the amount of drug the patient receives for a specific time. If a tablet or capsule is ordered, the drug should be dissolved in 30 ml of warm water, administered through the tube, and followed with extra water. This procedure ensures that the drug is in the stomach and not left in the tube.

Nasogastric Feeding Calculations

Tube feeding (TF) solutions, e.g., Ensure, Ensure Plus, Osmolite, Isomil, can be given in full strength (100% tube feeding) and in a percentage strength (diluted tube feeding). When a percentage strength of solution is ordered, the nurse calculates the amount of solution and water that should be given.

Caution:

- *Do not* mix medications in the entire tube feeding solution. Medications to be administered through a feeding tube should be diluted in 30 ml of water and followed with extra water.
- Time-released or sustain-released drugs *should not* be crushed and diluted in water. The drug could be absorbed immediately and could cause an adverse reaction.

Percent (%) of a solution indicates its strength. Percent is a portion of 100, e.g., 20% is 20 of 100 parts ($^{20}/_{100}$). To find percent, the basic formula, ratio and proportion, or fractional equation can be used with the following changes.

D: Desired percent.

H: On hand volume which is 100.

V: Desired total volume.

X: Unknown amount of solution.

EXAMPLES

Problem 1:   Mary Smith has been receiving intravenous fluids for 5 days. A nasogastric tube was inserted and 250 ml (cc) of 50% Ensure solution was ordered q4h × 6 (1 day). Calculate how much Ensure and water is needed to make 250 ml (50% solution).

Method: 50% solution is 50 in 100 parts.

$$\frac{D}{H} \frac{\text{desired \%}}{\text{on hand volume}} \times V \text{ (desired total volume)}$$

$$\frac{50}{100} \times 250 =$$

$$\frac{12500}{100} = 125 \text{ ml of Ensure}$$

$$H : V :: D : X$$
$$100 : 250 :: 50 : X$$
$$100 X = 12500$$
$$X = 125 \text{ ml of Ensure}$$

How much water should be added?

Total amount − Amount of TF = Amount of water
  250 ml − 125 ml = 125 ml

Answer: 125 ml of Ensure + 125 ml of water.

Problem 2: Three days later Mary Smith's tube feeding order was changed. She is to receive 250 ml (cc) of 70% Osmolite solution q6h.

How much Osmolite solution and water should be mixed to equal 250 ml?

Method: 70% solution is 70 in 100 parts.

$$\frac{D}{H} \times V =$$

$$\frac{70}{100} \times 250 =$$

$$\frac{17500}{100} = 175 \text{ ml of}$$
Osmolite

H : V :: D : X
100 : 250 :: 70 : X
100 X = 17500
X = 175 ml of
Osmolite

How much water should be added?

Total amount − Amount of TF = Amount of water
  250 ml − 175 ml = 75 ml

Answer: 175 ml of Osmolite + 75 ml of water.

Problem 3: A week later Mary Smith's tube feeding order was changed to 250 ml (cc) of 40% Ensure Plus. How much Ensure Plus and water should be mixed to equal 250 ml?

Method: 40% solution is 40 in 100 parts.

$$\frac{D}{H} \times V =$$

$$\frac{40}{100} \times 250 =$$

$$\frac{10000}{100} = 100 \text{ ml of}$$
Ensure Plus

H : V :: D : X
100 : 250 :: 40 : X
100 X = 10000
X = 100 ml of
Ensure Plus

How much water should be added?

Total amount − Amount of TF = Amount of water
  250 ml − 100 ml = 150 ml

Answer: 100 ml of Ensure Plus + 150 ml of water.

SUMMARY PRACTICE PROBLEMS

For each question, give the correct dosage that should be administered.

1. Order: propranolol/Inderal 40 mg.
Drug available: Inderal 10 mg per tablet.

2. Order: sulfisoxazole/Gantrisin 0.5 g.
Drug available: Gantrisin 250 mg per tablet.

3. Order: digoxin 0.5 mg.
Drug available: digoxin 0.25 mg per tablet.

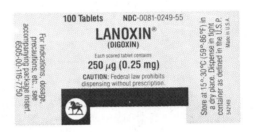

4. Order: codeine gr 1, PRN, q4h
Drug available:

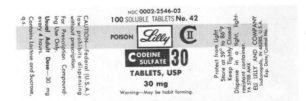

5. Order: ampicillin/Polycillin 0.5 g.
Drug available: ampicillin 250 mg per 5 ml.

6. Order: potassium chloride 40 mEq p.o.
Drug available: potassium chloride 20 mEq/15 ml.

7. Order: phenobarbital gr s̄s̄.
Drug available: phenobarbital 15 mg per tablet.

_____

8. Order: penicillin V suspension, 0.75 g.
Drug available: penicillin V 250 mg per 5 ml.

_____

9. Order: scopolamine gr $1/300$.
Drug available: scopolamine gr $1/150$ per 5 ml.

_____

10. Order: Mycostatin U 250,000 oral swish and swallow, qid.
Drug available: Mycostatin (oral suspension) u 100,000/ml.

_____

11. Order: diazepam/Valium 2½ mg.
Drug available: Valium 5 mg scored tablet.

_____

12. Order: hydrochlorothiazide/Hydro-DIURIL 0.1 g.
Drug available: Hydro-Diuril 50 mg tablet.

_____

13. Order: allopurinol 450 mg p.o. qd.
Drug available: allopurinol 300 mg scored tablet.

_____

14. Order: tolmetin sodium/Tolectin 400 mg.
Drug available: Tolectin 0.2 gm per tablet.

_____

15. Order: Valproic acid/Depakene 10 mg/kg/day in 3 divided doses (tid), p.o. Patient weighs 165 pounds. How much Depakene should be administered tid?

_____

16. Order: cyclophosphamide/Cytoxan 4 mg/kg/day p.o. Patient weighs 154 pounds. How much Cytoxan would you give per day?

_____

17. Order: mercaptopurine 2.5 mg/kg/day p.o. or 100 mg/m^2 body surface area p.o. The patient weighs 132 pounds and height is 64 inches. The estimated body surface area according to the nomogram is 1.7 m^2. The amount of drug the patient should receive according to kg is

_____ and according to m^2 is _____.

18. Order: 500 ml of 60% Ensure solution q8h through the nasogastric tube. How much Ensure solution and water should be mixed to equal 500 ml?

_____

19. Order: 250 ml of 80% Osmolite solution q6h through the nasogastric tube. How much Osmolite solution and water should be mixed to equal 250 ml?

_____

20. Order: 400 ml of 30% Ensure Plus solution q6h through the nasogastric tube. How much Ensure Plus solution and water should be mixed to equal 400 ml?

ANSWERS

1. $\dfrac{D}{H} \times V =$

    H : V :: D : X
    10 : 1 :: 40 : X

$\dfrac{40}{10} \times 1 =$

    10 X = 40
       X = 4 tablets

$\dfrac{40}{10} = 4$ tablets

2. 0.5 gm = 500 mg (Method A)

$\dfrac{D}{H} \times V = \dfrac{500}{250} \times 1 =$

    H : V :: D : X
    250 : 1 :: 500 : X

$\dfrac{500}{250} = 2$ tablets

    250 X = 500
       X = 2 tablets

3. 2 tablets.

4. 2 tablets. Change gr to mg. See a conversion table if needed.

5. 10 ml

6. 30 ml

7. Use the metric system. According to the conversion table in the appendix, gr ss = 30 mg.
   2 tablets

8. 15 ml

9. $\dfrac{D}{H} \times V = \dfrac{\frac{1}{300}}{\frac{1}{150}} \times 5 =$

$$H \; : \; V \; :: \; D \; : \; X$$
$$\tfrac{1}{150} \; : \; 5 \; :: \; \tfrac{1}{300} \; : \; X$$

$\dfrac{\frac{1}{300}}{\frac{1}{150}} \times 5 = \dfrac{5}{300} \times \dfrac{150}{1}$

$\dfrac{1}{150} X = \dfrac{5}{300}$

$X = \dfrac{5}{300} \times \dfrac{150}{1}$

$\dfrac{750}{300} = 2.5 \text{ ml}$

$X = \dfrac{750}{300}$

$X = 2.5 \text{ ml}$

10. $2\frac{1}{2}$ ml

11. $\frac{1}{2}$ tablet

12. 4 tablets

13. $1\frac{1}{2}$ tablets

14. 2 tablets

15. 165 lb = 75 kg (change pounds to kilograms by dividing 2.2 into the 165 pounds, 165 ÷ 2.2)

    10 mg × 75 = 750 mg
    750 ÷ 3 = 250 mg, tid.

16. 154 lb = 70 kg
    4 mg × 70 = 280 mg/day

17. 132 lb = 60 kg
    2.5 mg × 60 = 150 mg
    or
    100 × 1.7 = 170 mg

18. $\dfrac{D}{H} \times V = \dfrac{60}{100} \times 500 =$

    $$100 \; : \; 500 \; :: \; 60 \; : \; X$$
    $$100\,X = 30000$$

    $\dfrac{30000}{100} = 300 \text{ ml of Ensure}$

    $X = 300 \text{ ml of Ensure}$

    Total amount − Amount of TF = Amount of water
    500 ml − 300 ml = 200 ml

    300 ml of Ensure + 200 ml of water.

19. 200 ml of Osmolite + 50 ml of water

20. 120 ml of Ensure Plus + 280 ml of water

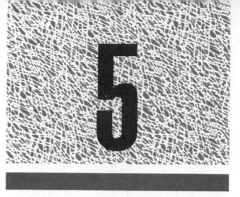

C H A P T E R

Injectable Preparations with Clinical Applications

Objectives

- Calculate dosage of drugs for subcutaneous and intramuscular routes from solutions in vials and ampules.
- Explain the procedure for preparing and calculating medications in powder form for injectable use.
- Determine prescribed insulin dosage in units using an insulin syringe.
- Explain the methods for mixing two insulin solutions in one insulin syringe and for mixing two injectable drugs in one syringe.
- Explain how to administer intradermal, subcutaneous, and intramuscular injections.
- Select correct syringe and needle for prescribed injectable drug.

Medications administered by injection may be given intradermally, subcutaneously (SC), or intramuscularly (IM). Injectable drugs are ordered in grams, milligrams, grains, and units. The preparations of injectable drugs may be packaged in a solvent (diluent or solution) or in a powder form.

This chapter provides information about syringes, needles, prefilled cartridges, vials, ampules, insulin preparation, and mixing drugs. Calculations for subcutaneous and intramuscular injections using drug solution and powder form of drugs are also included.

INJECTABLE PREPARATIONS

Vials and Ampules

Drugs are packaged in vials (sealed rubber-top containers) for single and multiple doses and in ampules (sealed glass containers) for a single dose. Multiple-dose vials may be used more than once because of the self-sealing rubber top; however, ampules are used only once after the glass neck container is opened. The drug is in either liquid or powder form in vials and ampules. When drugs in solution deteriorate rapidly, they are packaged in dry form and solvent (diluent) is added prior to administration.

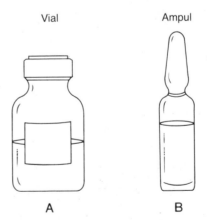

The route by which the injectable drug can be given, such as SC, IM, and/or IV, should be printed on the drug label.

Syringes and Needles

Types of syringes used for injections include 3 ml and 5 ml calibrated syringes, metal and plastic syringes for prefilled cartridges, tuberculin syringes, and insulin syringes. Occasionally a glass syringe may be used. Most glass syringes are used in the operating room and on special instrument trays.

An increasing number of injectable drugs are packaged in a prefilled cartridge with specified drug dose. The cartridge is placed into a Tubex syringe (metal or plastic holder) or Carpuject syringe (plastic syringe). The cartridge is disposed of after use. Usually a prefilled cartridge contains 0.1 to 0.2 ml of excess drug solution. The excess drug solution is given in case of accidental drug loss; however, if there is no loss, the excess solution must be expelled prior to administration.

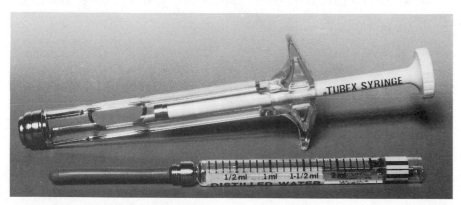

Courtesy of Wyeth Laboratories, Philadelphia, PA.

Needle size is determined by gauge (diameter of the lumen) and by length. The larger the gauge number, the smaller the diameter of the lumen. With a smaller gauge number, the diameter of the lumen is larger. The usual range of needle gauges is from 18 to 26. Needle length varies from ⅜ to 2 inches.

Needle sizes for subcutaneous and intradermal injections are:

1. small lumen: 23, 25, 26 gauge
2. needle lengths of ⅜, ½, ⅝ inch

Needle sizes for intramuscular injections are:

1. large lumen: 20, 21, 22 gauge
2. needle lengths of 1, 1 ½, and 2 inches

When choosing the length size for a patient receiving an intramuscular injection, the degree or amount of adipose tissue must be assessed.

Insulin syringes and prefilled cartridges have permanently attached needles. With other syringes, needle sizes can be changed. Needle gauge and length are indicated on the syringe package or the top cover of the syringe. It appears as gauge/length, such as 21 g/1 ½.

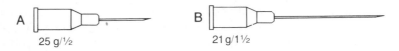

A 25 g/½   B 21 g/1½

Practice Problems

1. Which would have the larger needle lumen, a 21 gauge needle or a 25 gauge needle? _____.

2. Which would have the smaller needle lumen, an 18 gauge needle or a 26 gauge needle? _____.

3. Which needle would have a length of 1 ½ inches, a 20 gauge needle or a 25 gauge needle? _____.

4. Which needle would have a length of ⅝ inch, a 21 gauge needle or a 25 gauge needle? _____.

5. Which needle would be used for an intramuscular injection, a 21 gauge needle with a 1 ½ inch length or 25 gauge needle with a ⅝ inch length? _____.

ANSWERS

1. The 21 gauge needle, since it is the smaller gauge number.

2. The 26 gauge needle, since it is the larger gauge number.

3. The 20 gauge needle, since it has the larger lumen (small gauge). A needle with a 20 gauge and 1 ½ inch length is used for intramuscular injection.

4. The 25 gauge needle, since it has the smaller lumen (larger gauge). It would be used for subcutaneous injections. The length of the needle would not be long enough for an intramuscular injection.

5. The 21 gauge needle with 1 ½ inch length (21 g/1 ½). Muscle is under subcutaneous or fatty tissue, so a longer needle size is needed.

INTRADERMAL INJECTIONS

Usually an intradermal injection is used for skin testing for diagnostic purposes. Primary uses are for tuberculin and allergy testing. The tuberculin syringe (25 g/½ inch) holds 1 ml (16 minims) and is calibrated in 0.1 to 0.01 ml.

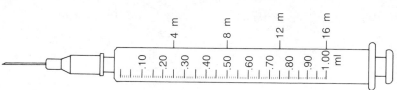

Tuberculin syringe

The skin area frequently chosen in skin testing is the inner aspect of the forearm, which has less hair. Test results would be more visible than on the hairy side of the forearm. The upper back may also be a testing site. The needle is inserted with the bevel upward at a 10 to 15 degree angle. Do not aspirate. Test results are usually read 48 hours after the intradermal injection. An induration (raised or thickened area) with erythema (redness) is a significant reaction.

SUBCUTANEOUS INJECTIONS

Drugs injected into the subcutaneous (fatty) tissue are absorbed slowly. This may be due to fewer blood vessels in fatty tissue. Doses of 0.5 to 1 ml of water-soluble drugs are indicated for subcutaneous injection and are administered at a 45 or 60 degree angle. Irritating solutions are usually given intramuscularly because they can cause sloughing of subcutaneous tissue.

Syringes that are primarily used for subcutaneous injections are the tuberculin syringe for dosages that require 0.5 ml or less (see tuberculin syringe), the 3 ml syringe, and the insulin syringe (discussed later). These syringes use a 26 or 25 gauge needle.

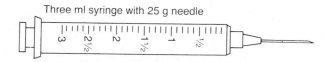

Three ml syringe with 25 g needle

Calculation for Subcutaneous Injections

Formulas for solving problems of subcutaneous injections are the basic formula of $\frac{D}{H} \times V$, ratio and proportion, and fractional equation (see Chapter 3). The following two problems are examples of injections that may be given subcutaneously.

EXAMPLES

Problem 1: Order: heparin U 5000, SC.

Drug available: heparin U 10,000/ml in multiple-dose (10 ml) vial.

Methods: *Basic Formula*   *Ratio and Proportion*

$$\frac{D}{H} \times V =$$

$$
\begin{array}{ccccccc}
H & : & V & :: & D & : & X \\
10,000 & : & 1 & :: & 5000 & : & X
\end{array}
$$

$$\frac{5000}{10000} \times 1 =$$ $$10,000\ X = 5000$$

$$\frac{5}{10} = 0.5 \text{ ml}$$ $$X = \frac{5000}{10000} = \frac{5}{10} = 0.5 \text{ ml}$$

Answer: Heparin U 5000 = 0.5 ml (use tuberculin syringe).

Problem 2:   Order: morphine 10 mg, SC.

Drug available:

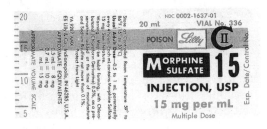

See label with approximate equivalents.

Methods: $$\frac{D}{H} \times V =$$

$$
\begin{array}{ccccccc}
H & : & V & :: & D & : & X \\
15 & : & 1 & :: & 10 & : & X
\end{array}
$$

$$\frac{10}{15} \times 1 =$$ $$15\ X = 10$$

$$\frac{2}{3} = 0.67 \text{ ml or} \atop 0.7 \text{ ml}$$ $$X = \frac{\overset{2}{\cancel{10}}}{\underset{3}{\cancel{15}}} = \frac{2}{3} = 0.67 \text{ ml or} \atop 0.7 \text{ ml}$$

Answer: Morphine 10 mg = 0.67 or 0.7 ml (use a tuberculin syringe or 3 ml syringe).

Practice Problems

Use the formula you chose for calculating oral drug dosages when solving Practice Problems 2, 3, 4, and 5.

1. Which needle gauge and length might be used for a subcutaneous injection, a 25 g/⅝ or 26 g/⅜? _____.

2. Order: heparin U 4000, SC.

Drug available: heparin U 10,000/ml in a multidose vial.

How many ml of heparin would you give?

_____

3. Order: heparin U 7500, SC.

Drug available: heparin U 10,000/ml in a multidose vial.

How many ml of heparin would you give?

_____

4. Order: atropine SO_4 gr $\frac{1}{100}$, SC.

Drug available:

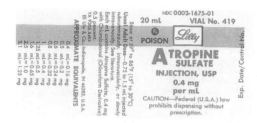

How many ml of atropine would you give?

_____

5. Order: epinephrine/Adrenalin 0.35 mg, SC, stat.

Drug available: epinephrine 1 mg (1:1000)/1 ml in ampule.

How many ml of epinephrine would you give? What type of syringe would you use? At what angle would you administer the drug?

ANSWERS

1. *Both* needle gauge and length could be used.

2. 0.4 ml

3. ¾ ml or 0.75 ml

4. Change grains (apothecary system) to mg (metric system). See Table 2–1: gr $\frac{1}{100}$ = 0.6 mg.

$$\frac{D}{H} \times V = \qquad\qquad \begin{array}{ccccccc} H & : & V & :: & D & : & X \\ 0.4 & : & 1 & :: & 0.6 & : & X \end{array}$$

$$\frac{0.6}{0.4} \times 1 = \qquad\qquad 0.4\,X = 0.6$$

$$\frac{0.6}{0.4} = 1.5 \text{ ml} \qquad\qquad X = \frac{0.6}{0.4} = 1.5 \text{ ml}$$

5. 0.35 ml of epinephrine; tuberculin syringe; 45 or 60 degree angle. The angle depends on the size of the subcutaneous tissue. For a thin person with less subcutaneous tissue, a 45 degree angle would probably be used.

INSULIN INJECTIONS

Insulin is prescribed and measured in USP units. Most insulins are manufactured in concentrations of 100 units per ml. Insulin should be administered with an insulin syringe, which is calculated to correspond with the U 100 insulin. Insulin bottles and syringes are color-coded. The U 100/ml insulin bottle and the U 100/ml syringe are color-coded orange. Insulin concentrations are also available in U 40 and U 500 but are not commonly used. U 40 will be phased out by the FDA and U 500 is used mainly in acute situations.

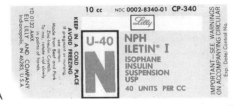

A

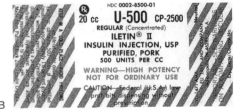

B

The insulin syringe may be marked with one side in even units (10, 20, 30, etc.) and the other side in odd units (5, 15, 25, etc.).

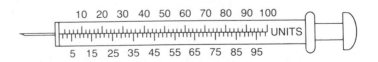

Actually, insulin is easy to prepare and administer as long as the nurse uses the *same insulin concentration with the same calibrated insulin syringe*, e.g., a U 100 per ml insulin bottle and a U 100 per ml insulin syringe. If the prescribed insulin dosage is 30 units, withdraw 30 units from a bottle of U 100 insulin using a U 100 calibrated insulin syringe. Administering insulin with a tuberculin syringe is NOT suggested and DEFINITELY SHOULD BE AVOIDED.

Types of Insulin

1. Fast-acting (Humulin, crystalline or regular, and Semilente)

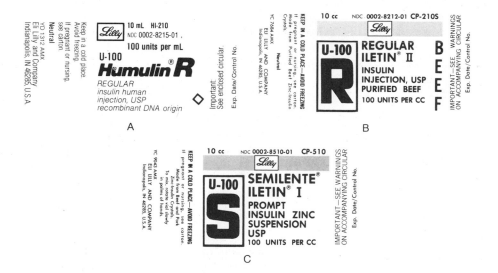

A   B

C

2. Intermediate-acting (Humulin, NPH, and Lente)

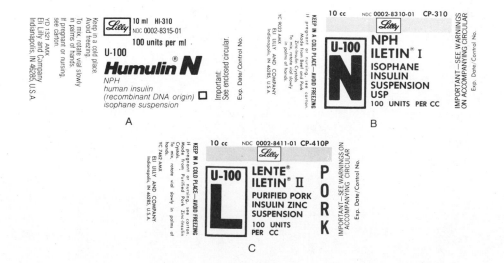

A   B

C

3. Long-acting (PZI and Ultralente)

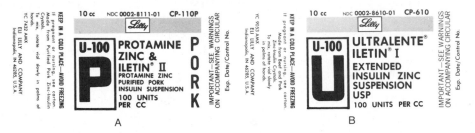

A

B

Regular insulin is clear and is the only type of insulin that can be given intravenously as well as subcutaneously. All other insulins are cloudy owing to the protamine and zinc, and thus can be administered only subcutaneously.

Insulin is administered subcutaneously at a 45 or 60 or 90 degree angle into the subcutaneous tissue. The angle for administering insulin depends upon the amount of fatty tissue. For a very thin person, the 45 degree angle is suggested. The 90 degree angle should be used on obese or average-sized persons. When using the 90 degree angle, pinch the skin upward so the insulin is deposited into the fatty tissue.

Mixing Insulins

Regular insulin is frequently mixed with insulins containing protamine, such as NPH, and zinc, such as Lente. The protamine and zinc in insulins prolong the duration of action. The source of insulin is beef, pork, beef-pork, and human (Humulin). Some persons are allergic to beef insulin, so pork insulin is used because it has biologic properties similar to human insulin.

EXAMPLE: Problem and method for mixing insulin.

Problem 1: Order: Regular insulin 10 units and Lente insulin 40 units, SC.

Drug available: Regular insulin U 100/ml and Lente insulin U 100/ml, both in multidose vials. The insulin syringe is marked U 100/ml.

Methods: **1.** Cleanse the rubber tops or diaphragms of insulin bottles.

2. Draw up 40 units of air and inject into the Lente insulin bottle. Avoid the needle's coming into contact with the Lente insulin solution. Withdraw needle.

3. Draw up 10 units of air and inject into the regular insulin bottle.

4. Withdraw 10 units of regular insulin. Regular insulin is withdrawn before Lente and NPH.

5. Withdraw 40 units of Lente insulin.

6. Administer the two insulins immediately after mixing. Do NOT allow the insulin mixture to stand because unpredicted physical changes might occur. Unpredicted changes are more common with protamine insulins such as NPH and PZI than with Lente insulin.

Practice Problems

1. Order: NPH insulin 35 units, SC.

Drug available: NPH insulin U 100/ml and U 100/ml insulin syringe.

How much insulin would you withdraw?

_____

2. Order: Lente insulin 50 units, SC.

Drug available: Lente U 100/ml and U 100/ml insulin syringe.

How much insulin would you withdraw?

_____

3. Order: Regular insulin 8 units and NPH insulin 52 units.

Drug available: Regular insulin U 100/ml and NPH insulin U 100/ml. The insulin syringe is U 100/ml.

Explain the method for mixing the two insulins.

Mark on the U 100/ml insulin syringe how much regular insulin should be withdrawn and how much NPH insulin should be withdrawn.

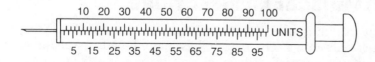

_____

4. Order: regular insulin 15 units and Lente insulin 45 units

Drug available: Regular insulin U 100/ml and Lente insulin U 100/ml. The insulin syringe is U 100/ml.

Explain the method for mixing the two insulins.

Mark on the U 100/ml insulin syringe how much regular insulin and how much Lente insulin should be withdrawn.

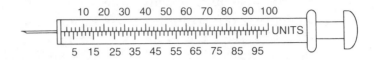

ANSWERS

1. Withdraw 35 units of NPH insulin to the 35 mark on the insulin syringe. Both the insulin and the syringe have the same concentration, U 100/ml.

2. Withdraw 50 units of Lente insulin to the 50 mark on the insulin syringe. Both the insulin and the syringe have the same concentration, U 100/ml.

3. Inject 52 units of air into the NPH insulin bottle. Do not allow the needle to touch the insulin solution. Inject 8 units of air into the regular insulin bottle and withdraw 8 units of regular insulin. Withdraw 52 units of NPH insulin. Total amount of insulin should be 60 units. Do NOT allow the insulin mixture to stand. Administer immediately, since NPH contains protamine and unpredicted physical changes could result.

4. Inject 45 units of air into the Lente insulin bottle. Inject 15 units of air into the regular insulin bottle and withdraw 15 units of regular insulin. Withdraw 45 units of Lente insulin. Total amount of insulin should be 60 units. Insulin mixture may stand for a short period of time since it is Lente insulin.

INTRAMUSCULAR INJECTIONS

The intramuscular (IM) injection is a common method of administering injectable drugs. The muscle has many blood vessels (more so than fatty tissue), so medications given by intramuscular injections are absorbed more rapidly than subcutaneous injections. The volume of solution for an IM injection is 0.5 to 3.0 ml with the average being 1 to 2 ml. A volume of drug solution greater than 3 ml causes increased muscle tissue displacement and possible tissue damage. Occasionally 5 ml of certain drugs, such as magnesium sulfate, may be injected in a large muscle such as the dorsogluteal. Dosage greater than 3 ml is usually split between two sites.

Syringes used for intramuscular injections are 3 ml and 5 ml syringes, prefilled cartridge for metal or plastic syringe, and tuberculin (TB) syringe. The tuberculin syringe may be used to administer a drug solution intramuscularly when ½ ml (0.5 ml) or less is needed. The needle on the tuberculin syringe (25 g/½ inch) would be changed to a 20–22 g/1–2 inches for IM injections.

Examples of 3 ml and 5 ml syringes are:

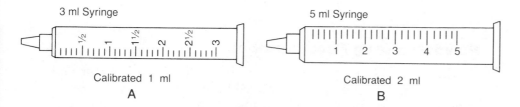

Intramuscular injections are administered at a 90 degree angle. The needle length depends upon the degree or amount of adipose and muscle tissue; thus, needle length is a judgment of the nurse.

The average needle length is 1 ½ inches.

EXAMPLES

Two problems are given as examples for calculating IM dosage. Choose one of the three methods for calculating drug dosage.

Problem 1: Order: gentamycin 60 mg, IM.

Drug available: gentamycin 80 mg/2 ml in a vial.

Methods:

$$\frac{D}{H} \times V =$$

$$\frac{60}{80} \times 2 =$$

$$\frac{120}{80} = 1.5 \text{ ml}$$

$$
\begin{array}{ccccccc}
H & : & V & :: & D & : & X \\
80 & : & 2 & :: & 60 & : & X
\end{array}
$$

$$80 X = 120$$

$$X = \frac{120}{80} = 1.5 \text{ ml}$$

Answer: Gentamycin 60 mg = 1.5 ml.

Problem 2: Order: lanoxin/Digoxin 0.15 mg, IM.

Drug available:

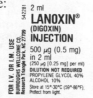

542281 2 ml
LANOXIN®
(DIGOXIN)
INJECTION
500 µg (0.5 mg)
in 2 ml
(250 µg [0.25 mg] per ml)
DILUTION NOT REQUIRED
PROPYLENE GLYCOL 40%
ALCOHOL 10%
Store at 15°–30°C (59°–86°F).
Protect from light.
FOR I.V. OR I.M. USE
BURROUGHS WELLCOME CO.
Research Triangle Park, NC 27709
LOT
EXP.

Methods:

$$\frac{D}{H} \times V =$$

$$H \quad : \quad V \quad :: \quad D \quad : \quad X$$
$$0.5 \quad : \quad 2 \quad :: \quad 0.15 \quad : \quad X$$

$$\frac{0.15}{0.5} \times 2 = \qquad\qquad 0.5\,X = 0.30$$

$$\frac{0.30}{0.5} = 0.6 \text{ ml} \qquad\qquad X = \frac{0.30}{0.5} = 0.6 \text{ ml}$$

Answer: Lanoxin/Digoxin 0.15 mg = 0.6 ml.

Powdered Drug Reconstitution

Certain drugs lose their potency in liquid form. Therefore, manufacturers package these drugs in powdered form and they are reconstituted prior to administration. To reconstitute a drug, look on the drug label or in the instructional insert (circular pamphlet) for the type and amount of diluent to use. Sterile water, bacteriostatic water, and normal saline are the primary diluents. If the type and amount of diluent are not on the drug label or in the instructional insert, then call the pharmacy.

The powdered drug occupies space and therefore increases the volume of drug solution. Usually manufacturers determine the amount of diluent to mix with the drug powder to yield 1 to 2 ml per desired dose. Once the powdered drug has been reconstituted, the unused drug solution should be dated, refrigerated, and initialed. Most drugs retain their potency for 96 hours to one week when refrigerated. Check the drug circular or drug label for how long the reconstituted drug may be used.

EXAMPLES

Three problems are given as examples for mixing drugs in powdered form for intramuscular injections. With Problem 3, the amount of diluent is not printed on the drug label.

Problem 1:   Order: aqueous penicillin U 500,000, IM.

Drug available:

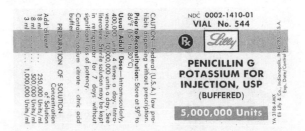

According to the label on the bottle, the amount of pow-dered drug in the vial is U 5,000,000 (5 million units). The drug label states:

Diluent Added	Units per ml
18 ml	250,000
*8 ml	500,000
3 ml	1,000,000

Add 8 ml of diluent. The drug powder is equivalent to 2 ml. Each U 500,000 equals 1 ml.

Methods:

$$\frac{D}{H} \times V =$$

$$H \quad : \quad V \quad : : \quad D \quad : \quad X$$
$$5,000,000 \quad : \quad 10 \quad : : \quad 500,000 \quad : \quad X$$

$$\frac{500,000}{5,000,000} \times 10 = \qquad\qquad 50\,X = 50$$

$$\frac{50}{50} = 1 \text{ ml} \qquad\qquad X = 1 \text{ ml}$$

Answer: Aq. penicillin U 500,000 = 1 ml.

Problem 2: Order: cefazolin/Kefzol 500 mg, IM.

Drug available:

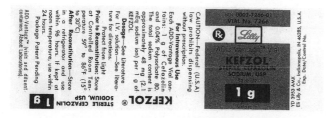

The drug literature reads to add 4 ml of sterile water, and 0.5 g = 2.2 ml.

Answer: Cefazolin/Kefzol 500 mg = 2.2 ml.

Problem 3: Order: cefoxitin/Mefoxin 250 mg, IM.

Drug available: The drug label indicates that the vial contains 1 g Mefoxin. When manufacturers assume that the entire drug will be used, they may not print the type and amount of diluent on the drug label or literature insert (circular pamphlet).

If only a portion of the drug is needed:

1. Mix the entire drug with a diluent. Because the amount of diluent is not given, you could add 2 ml, 4 ml, 6 ml, 8 ml, or 10 ml. Remember not to give more than 2½ ml at one site. Since you will use ¼ of the drug in the vial, you *may* add 4 ml of diluent.

2. Withdraw the dissolved solution to determine the total volume of solution (diluent plus powder drug). The total volume of Mefoxin solution is 4.5 ml. Inject the fluid back into the vial.

3. Calculate the amount of solution for the prescribed drug dose from the total drug volume. Use one of the formulas in calculating drug dosage.

4. Withdraw the drug volume for the prescribed dose.

Methods: Change grams to milligrams by moving the decimal point three places to the right: 1 g = 1.000 mg.

$$\frac{D}{H} \times V = \qquad H \quad : \quad V \quad :: \quad D \quad : \quad X$$
$$\phantom{\frac{D}{H} \times V =} \qquad 1000 \text{ mg} \ : \ 4.5 \ :: \ 250 \text{ mg} \ : \ X$$

$$\frac{250}{1000} \times 4.5 = \qquad\qquad 1000 \, X = 1125$$

$$\frac{1125}{1000} = 1.1 \text{ ml} \qquad\qquad X = 1.12 \text{ ml or}$$
$$\phantom{\frac{1125}{1000} = 1.1 \text{ ml} \qquad\qquad X =} 1.1 \text{ ml}$$

Answer: Mefoxin 250 mg = 1.1 ml.

Mixing Injectable Drugs

Drugs mixed together in the same syringe must be compatible to prevent precipitation. To determine drug compatibility, check drug references or check with a pharmacist. When in doubt of compatibility, do NOT mix drugs.

Method 1: Mixing two drugs in the same syringe from *two vials.*

1. Draw air in syringe to equal the amount of solution to be withdrawn from the first vial and inject the air into the first vial. Do NOT allow the needle to come into contact with the solution. Remove the needle.

2. Draw air in syringe to equal the amount of solution to be withdrawn from the second vial. Invert second vial and inject the air.

3. Withdraw the desired amount of solution from the second vial.

4. Change the needle unless you will use the entire volume in the first vial.

5. Invert first vial and withdraw the desired amount of solution.

or

1. Draw air in syringe to equal the amount of solution to be withdrawn and inject the air into the first vial. Withdraw the desired drug dose.

2. Insert a 25 g needle in the rubber-top vial (not in the center) of the second vial. This acts as an air vent. Injecting air into the second vial is NOT necessary.

3. Insert the needle in the center of the rubber-top vial (beside the 25 g needle-air vent), invert second vial and withdraw the desired drug dose.

Method 2:   Mixing two drugs in the same syringe from *one vial and one ampule.*

1. Remove the amount of desired solution from the vial.

2. Aspirate the amount of desired solution from the ampule.

Method 3:   Mixing two drugs in a *prefilled cartridge from a vial.*

1. Check the drug dose and the amount of solution in the prefilled cartridge. If a smaller dose is needed, expel the excess solution.

2. Draw air into the cartridge to equal the amount of solution to be withdrawn from the vial. Invert the vial and inject the air.

3. Withdraw desired amount of solution from the vial. Make sure the needle remains in the fluid and do NOT take more solution than needed.

EXAMPLES: Mixing drugs in the same syringe.

Problem 1:   Order: meperidine/Demerol 60 mg and atropine SO_4 gr $\frac{1}{150}$, IM. The two drugs are compatible.

Drug available: meperidine in a Tubex cartridge labeled 100 mg/ml. Atropine SO_4 in a multidose vial labeled 0.4 mg/ml (mg/ml means mg/l ml).

How many ml of each drug would you give?

Explain how to mix the two drugs.

Methods: *Meperidine* 100 mg/ml.

$$\frac{D}{H} \times V =$$

$$H \quad : \quad V \quad :: \quad D \quad : \quad X$$
$$100 \quad : \quad 1 \quad :: \quad 60 \quad : \quad X$$

$$\frac{60}{100} \times 1 = 0.6 \text{ ml}$$

$$100 \text{ X} = 60$$
$$X = 0.6 \text{ ml}$$

Atropine SO$_4$

gr $\frac{1}{150}$ = 0.4 mg (see Table 2–1 or conversion table in Appendix B)

Answer: Meperidine/Demerol 60 mg = 0.6 ml.
Atropine gr $\frac{1}{150}$ = 1 ml.

Procedure: Mix two drugs in cartridge with one drug from a vial.

1. Check drug dose and volume on prefilled cartridge.

2. Expel 0.4 ml and any excess of drug solution from cartridge; 0.6 ml remains in the cartridge.

3. Draw 1 ml of air in the cartridge and inject into vial.

4. Withdraw 1 ml of drug solution from vial into the prefilled cartridge.

Problem 2:   Pre-op order: meperidine 25 mg, Vistaril 25 mg, and Robinul 0.1 mg. All three drugs are compatible.

Drug available: meperidine/Demerol is in a 2 ml Tubex cartridge labeled 50 mg/ml. Hydroxyzine/Vistaril, 50 mg/ml ampule. Glycopyrrolate/Robinul, 0.2 mg/ml vial.

How many ml of each drug would you give?

Explain how the drugs could be mixed together.

Methods: **a.** Meperidine 25 mg. Label: 50 mg/ml.

$$\frac{D}{H} \times V =$$

$$H \quad : \quad V \quad :: \quad D \quad : \quad X$$
$$50 \quad : \quad 1 \quad :: \quad 25 \quad : \quad X$$

$$\frac{25}{50} \times 1 = 0.5 \text{ ml}$$

$$50 \text{ X} = 25$$
$$X = \frac{1}{2} \text{ ml or } 0.5 \text{ ml}$$

b. Vistaril 25 mg. Label: 50 mg/ml ampule.

$$\frac{D}{H} \times V =$$

$$H \quad : \quad V \quad :: \quad D \quad : \quad X$$
$$50 \quad : \quad 1 \quad :: \quad 25 \quad : \quad X$$

$$\frac{25}{50} \times 1 = 0.5 \text{ ml}$$

$$50 \text{ X} = 25$$
$$X = \frac{1}{2} \text{ ml or } 0.5 \text{ ml}$$

c. Robinul 0.1 mg. Label 0.2 mg/ml.

$$\frac{D}{H} \times V =$$

$$H \ : \ V \ :: \ D \ : \ X$$
$$0.2 \ : \ 1 \ :: \ 0.1 \ : \ X$$

$$\frac{0.1}{0.2} \times 1 = 0.5 \ ml$$

$$0.2 \ X = 0.1$$
$$X = 0.5 \ ml$$

Answer: Meperidine/Demerol 25 mg = 0.5 ml;
Vistaril 25 mg = 0.5 ml; Robinul 0.1 mg = 0.5 ml.

Procedure: Mix the three drugs in the cartridge.

1. Check drug dose and volume on prefilled cartridge. Expel 0.5 ml of meperidine and any excess of drug solution from cartridge.
2. Draw 0.5 ml of air in the cartridge and inject in the vial containing the Robinul.
3. Withdraw 0.5 ml of Robinul from the vial into the prefilled cartridge containing meperidine.
4. Withdraw 0.5 ml of Vistaril from the ampule into the cartridge.

Calculation of Injectables by Body Weight

Medications may be ordered for injections based on body weight. Review sections on body weight in Chapters 3 and 4.

EXAMPLE:

Problem: Order: Netilmicin SO_4/Netromycin 2.0 mg/kg, q8h, IM.

The patient weighs 174 pounds.

Drug available: netilmicin 100 mg/ml.

How many ml would you give q8h?

Method: **a.** Convert pounds to kilograms; 2.2 lb = 1 kg.

$$174 \div 2.2 = 79.1 \ kg$$

b. 2 mg × 79.1 = 158 mg q8h.

c.
$$\frac{D}{H} \times V =$$

$$H \ : \ V \ :: \ D \ : \ X$$
$$100 \ : \ 1 \ :: \ 158 \ : \ X$$

$$\frac{158}{100} \times 1 =$$

$$100 \ X = 158$$
$$X = 1.58 \ or \ 1.6 \ ml$$

1.58 or 1.6 ml

Answer: Netilmicin 2.0 mg/kg = 1.6 ml.

Practice Problems

1. Order: prochlorperazine/Compazine 8 mg, IM, stat.

   Drug available: 10 mg/2 ml in vial.

   How many milliliters (ml) would you give?

   _____

2. Order: methylprednisolone/Solu-Medrol 75 mg, IM, qd.

   Drug available: 125 mg/2 ml in vial.

   How many ml would you give?

   _____

3. Order: cyanocobalamin/Rubramin 125 mcg, IM, qd.

   Drug available: 100 mcg (microgram)/ml

   How many ml would you give?

   _____

4. Order: Narcan 0.2 mg, IM, stat.

   Drug available: 0.4 mg/ml in ampule.

   How many ml would you give?

   _____

5. Order: meperidine/Demerol 35 mg and promethazine/Phenergan 10 mg, IM.

   Drug available: meperidine 50 mg/ml prefilled cartridge, which can hold 2 ml of solution (2 ml cartridge). Promethazine 25 mg/ml in ampule.

   How many ml of meperidine would you give? How many ml of promethazine?

   Explain how the two drugs would be mixed in the cartridge.

   _____

6. Order: meperidine/Demerol 50 mg and hydroxyzine/Vistaril 25 mg, IM. These two drugs are compatible.

   Drug available: meperidine 50 mg/ml in prefilled cartridge of 2 ml size. Hydroxyzine 100 mg/2 ml in vial.

   How many ml of meperidine and how many ml of hydroxyzine would you give?

   Explain how the two drugs would be mixed in the cartridge.

   _____

7. Order: cephalothin/Keflin 250 mg, IM, q8h.

Drug available:

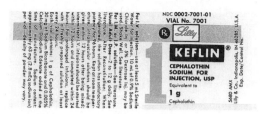

Literature insert reads to add 2.5 ml of diluent.

Total solution = 3 ml.

Change grams to milligrams.

How many ml of Keflin would you give every 8 hours?

How should this drug be labeled?

8. Order: procaine penicillin U 400,000, IM, q12h.

Drug available: procaine penicillin U 300,000/ml in white liquid form in a multiple-dose vial.

How many ml of procaine penicillin would you withdraw?

9. Order: ampicillin/Polycillin-N 400 mg, IM, q6h.

Drug available:

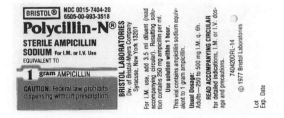

Drug label reads to add 3.5 ml of diluent. Total volume of solution would = 4.0 ml (1 g = 4 ml).

How many ml of ampicillin should be withdrawn?

10. Order: amikacin 15 mg/kg/day, q8h, IM.

Drug available:

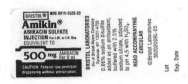

Patient weighs 140 pounds.

a. How many kg does the patient weigh?

_____

b. How many mg should the patient receive daily?

_____

c. How many mg should the patient receive q8h (three divided doses)

_____

d. How many ml should the patient receive q8h?

_____

ANSWERS

1. $\dfrac{D}{H} \times V =$

$\dfrac{8}{10} \times 2 =$

$\dfrac{16}{10} = 1.6$ ml

H : V :: D : X
10 : 2 :: 8 : X

10 X = 16
X = 1.6 ml

Give 1.6 ml of prochlorperazine IM.

2. 1.2 ml of Solu-Medrol.

3. 1.25 ml of Rubramin.

4. 0.5 ml of Narcan.

5. Meperidine 35 mg = 0.7 ml; promethazine 10 mg = 0.4 ml.

Procedure: **1.** Check meperidine dose and volume in prefilled cartridge.

2. Expel 0.3 ml and any excess in prefilled cartridge; 0.7 ml of solution should remain.

3. Withdraw 0.4 ml of promethazine from ampule into cartridge.

6. Meperidine 50 mg = 1 ml; hydroxyzine 25 mg = 0.5 ml.

  Procedure: **1.** Check meperidine dose and volume in prefilled cartridge.

           2. Expel any excess solution in prefilled cartridge; 1 ml of solution should remain.

           3. Draw 0.5 ml of air into cartridge and inject into vial.

           4. Withdraw 0.5 ml of hydroxyzine from vial into cartridge.

7. Change grams to milligrams by moving the decimal point three places to the right: 1.000 g = 1000 mg.
Keflin 250 mg = 0.75 ml.

8. 1.3 ml of procaine penicillin.

9. Change grams to milligrams; 1.000 g = 1000 mg.

$$\frac{D}{H} \times V = \qquad\qquad \text{H} \quad : \quad \text{V} \quad :: \quad \text{D} \quad : \quad \text{X}$$
$$\qquad\qquad\qquad 1000 \quad : \quad 4 \quad :: \quad 400 \quad : \quad \text{X}$$

$$\frac{400}{1000} \times 4 = \qquad\qquad 1000\ \text{X} = 1600$$

$$\frac{1600}{1000} = 1.6\ \text{ml} \qquad\qquad \text{X} = \frac{1600}{1000} = 1.6\ \text{ml}$$

Ampicillin 400 mg = 1.6 ml.

10. a. 140 ÷ 2.2 = 63.6 kg

   b. 15 mg × 63.6 × 1 = 954 mg daily

   c. 954 ÷ 3 = 318 mg of amikacin q8h

   d. $\dfrac{D}{H} \times V =$ H : V :: D : X
                               500 : 2 :: 318 : X

$$\frac{318}{500} \times 2 = \qquad\qquad 500\ \text{X} = 636$$
$$\qquad\qquad\qquad\qquad\qquad \text{X} = 1.27 \text{ or } 1.3 \text{ ml}$$

$$\frac{636}{500} = 1.27 \text{ or } 1.3 \text{ ml}$$

Give 1.27 or *1.3 ml* of amikacin q8h (three times a day).

CONTINUOUS INTRAVENOUS ADMINISTRATION

Intravenous Sets

Calculation of IV Flow Rate

Safety Considerations

Mixing Drugs Used for Continuous IV Administration

INTERMITTENT INTRAVENOUS ADMINISTRATION

Secondary IV Sets Without Controllers

Intermittent Infusion Adapters (Heparin Lock)

Electronic IV Regulators

Calculating Flow Rates for IV Drugs

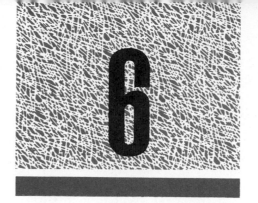

Intravenous Preparations with Clinical Applications

Objectives

- Examine the 3 methods for calculating intravenous (IV) flow rate and select one of the methods for IV calculation.
- Calculate drops per minute of prescribed intravenous solutions for IV therapy.
- Determine the drop factor according to manufacturer's product specification.
- Calculate the drug dosage for intravenous medications.
- Calculate flow rate for intravenous drugs being administered in a prescribed amount of solution.
- Explain the types and uses of IV electronic intravenous regulators.

Intravenous (IV) infusion is used in administering fluids and drugs. Two methods of administration are continuous IV infusion and intermittent IV infusion. Continuous IV administration replaces fluid loss, maintains fluid balance, and allows drug administration. Intermittent IV administration is primarily used for giving IV drugs.

Advantages for intravenous drugs are (1) rapid drug distribution into the bloodstream and (2) no drug loss to tissues. The disadvantage in giving drugs intravenously is that there is less time for corrective measures because the drug action is more rapid than if given subcutaneously or intramuscularly.

Nurses play an important role in preparing and administering intravenous solutions and drugs. The nursing functions and responsibilities include (1) knowledge of intravenous sets and their drop factors, (2) calculating IV flow rates, (3) mixing drugs and diluting in IV solution, and (4) regulating IV controllers.

CONTINUOUS INTRAVENOUS ADMINISTRATION

When intravenous (IV) solutions are required, the physician orders the amount of solution per liter or milliliters to be administered for a time period, such as for 24 hours. The nurse calculates the IV flow rate according to the drop factor, the amount of fluids to be administered, and the time period.

Intravenous Sets

There are various IV infusion sets. The drop factor, the number of drops per 1 milliliter, is usually printed on the package. Sets that deliver large drops per milliliter (10–20 gtts/ml) are referred to as macrodrip sets, and those with small drops per milliliter (60 gtts/ml) are called microdrip or minidrip sets.

Examples of sets that deliver macrodrip, large drops, are:

Manufacturer	Drops (gtts) per ml
Cutter	20 gtts/ml
Abbott	15 gtts/ml
McGaw	15 gtts/ml
Travenol	10 gtts/ml

All *microdrip sets* deliver *60 gtts per ml*. Check the box or package of the intravenous set used in your institution to determine the drop factor (gtts per ml). This is needed information to calculate and regulate IV flow rate. In most instances, the nurse has a choice to use either the macro-drip or microdrip set. If the IV rate is to infuse at 100 ml/hr or more, the macrodrip sets are recommended. For rates less than 100 ml/hr, the microdrip set is usually used. Low rates make macrodrip adjustment tedious; for example, for 50 ml/hr, the macrodrip rate would be 8 gtts/minute.

Calculation of IV Flow Rate

Three different methods may be used to calculate IV flow rate (drops per minute or gtts/min). The nurse should select one of the methods, memorize it, and use it to calculate dosages.

Method I: Three-step

$$\textbf{a.}\ \frac{\text{Amount of solution}}{\text{Hours to administer}} = \text{ml/hr}$$

$$\textbf{b.}\ \frac{\text{ml per hour}}{60\ \text{minutes}} = \text{ml/min}$$

c. ml per minute $\times$ gtts per ml = gtts/min
of IV set

Method II: Two-step (a frequently chosen method)

a. Amount of fluid $\div$ hours to administer = ml/hr

$$\textbf{b.}\ \frac{\text{ml per hour} \times \text{gtts per ml (IV set)}}{60\ \text{minutes}} = \text{gtts/min}$$

Method III: One-step

$$\frac{\text{Amount of fluid} \times \text{gtts per ml (IV set)}}{\text{Hours to administer} \times \text{minutes per hour (60)}} = \text{gtts/min}$$

Safety Considerations

All IV infusions should be checked every hour to ensure the rate of infusion and to assess for potential problems. Common problems asso-ciated with IV infusions are kinked tubing, extravasation of IV fluids, and "runaway" IV rates. IVs using electronic intravenous regulators need to be monitored. Mechanical problems or incorrect settings may cause incorrect fluid administration. Fluid overload, thrombus formation, and infiltration at the IV site are complications of IV therapy that can be avoided with frequent monitoring of the IV infusion.

At times intravenous fluids are given at a slow rate to *keep vein open* (KVO), also called *to keep open* (TKO). The purposes for ordering KVO might be (1) for a suspected emergency situation so that fluids and drugs could be quickly administered and (2) as an open line to give IV drugs every so many hours. For KVO, a microdrip set (60 gtts/min) and a 250 ml IV bag may be used. The suggested ml/hr is usually 10 ml/hr for 24 hours.

Mixing Drugs Used for Continuous IV Administration

Drugs such as multiple vitamins and potassium chloride may be added to the intravenous solution bag for continuous IV infusion. It is suggested that the drug(s) be added to the bag or bottle immediately before administering the intravenous fluid. Inject the drug into the rubber stopper on the IV bag or bottle and rotate several times to ensure dispersal of the drug. Do NOT add the drug while the infusion is running unless the bag is rotated.

If drugs are injected into an IV bag prior to use, the bag should not sit for hours unless it is refrigerated. Refrigeration maintains drug potency.

EXAMPLES

Two problems for determining IV flow rate are given. Each problem is solved using the three methods for calculating IV flow rate.

Problem 1: Order: 1000 ml of 5% D/½ NSS (5% dextose in ½ normal saline solution) in 6 hours.

Available: 1 liter (1000 ml) of D_5/½ NSS solution bag. IV set labeled 10 gtts/ml.

How many drops per minute should the patient receive?

Method I: **a.** $\dfrac{1000 \text{ ml}}{6 \text{ hr}} = 166.6$ or 167 ml/hr

b. $\dfrac{167 \text{ ml}}{60 \text{ min}} = 2.7$ or 2.8 ml/min

c. 2.8 ml/min $\times$ 10 gtts/ml = 28 gtts/min

Method II: **a.** 1000 ml ÷ 6 hr = 167 ml/hr

b. $\dfrac{167 \text{ ml/hr} \times \overset{1}{\cancel{10}} \text{ gtts/ml}}{\underset{6}{\cancel{60}} \text{ min}} = \dfrac{167}{6} = 28$ gtts/min

10 and 60 cancel to 1 and 6.

If ml/hr is given, use only the b portion of the method for calculating IV flow rate.

Method III:
$$\frac{1000 \text{ ml} \times \overset{1}{\cancel{10}} \text{ gtts/ml}}{6 \text{ hr} \times \underset{6}{\cancel{60}} \text{ min}} = \frac{1000}{36} = 27\text{--}28 \text{ gtts/min}$$

10 and 60 cancel to 1 and 6.

The use of a hand calculator is highly suggested to avoid errors.

Answer: 28 gtts/min.

Problem 2: Order: 1000 ml of D_5W (5% dextrose in water), 1 vial of MVI (multiple vitamin), and 20 mEq of KCl (potassium chloride) every 8 hours.

Available: 1000 ml D_5W solution bag
1 vial of MVI = 5 ml
40 mEq/20 ml of KCl in an ampule
IV set labeled 15 gtts/ml

How many ml of KCl would you withdraw to be equivalent to 20 mEq of KCl?

How would you mix KCl in the IV bag?

How many gtts/min?

Procedure: MVI: Inject 5 ml of MVI into the rubber stopper on the IV bag.

KCl: Calculate the prescribed dosage for KCl using the basic formula or ratio and proportion.

$$\frac{D}{H} \times V = \qquad \begin{array}{ccccccc} H & : & V & :: & D & : & X \\ 40 & : & 20 & :: & 20 & : & X \end{array}$$

$$\frac{20}{40} \times 20 = \qquad \begin{array}{c} 40 \text{ X} = 400 \\ \text{X} = 10 \text{ ml} \end{array}$$

$$\frac{400}{40} = 10 \text{ ml}$$

Withdraw 10 ml of KCl and inject into the rubber stopper on the IV bag. Make sure the KCl solution is dispersed throughout the IV bag by rotating the IV bag.

Method I: a. $\dfrac{1000 \text{ ml}}{8 \text{ hr}} = 125 \text{ ml/hr}$

b. $\dfrac{125 \text{ ml}}{60 \text{ min}} = 2.0\text{-}2.1 \text{ ml/min}$

c. $2.1 \times 15 = 31\text{-}32 \text{ gtts/min}$

Method II: **a.** $1000 \div 8 = 125 \text{ ml/hr}$

b. $\dfrac{125 \text{ ml/hr} \times \overset{1}{\cancel{15}} \text{ gtts/ml}}{\underset{4}{\cancel{60} \text{ min}}} = \dfrac{125}{4} = 31\text{-}32 \text{ gtts/min}$

15 and 60 cancel to 1 and 4.

IV flow rate should be 31 to 32 gtts/min.

Method III: $\dfrac{1000 \text{ ml} \times \overset{1}{\cancel{15}} \text{ gtts/ml}}{\underset{4}{8 \text{ hr} \times \cancel{60} \text{ min}}} = \dfrac{1000}{32} = 32 \text{ gtts/min}$

15 and 60 cancel to 1 and 4.

IV flow rate should be 31 to 32 gtts/min.

NOTE: The amount of IV fluid may include the volume of the drug added to the IV. This may be important for patients on strict I & O. The amount of fluid used in this problem was 1000 ml; however, it could be 1015 ml (1000 ml + 15 ml for KCl and MVI).

Answer: 32 gtts/min.

Practice Problems

Select *one* of the three methods for calculating IV flow rate.

1. Order: 1000 ml of D_5W to run for 12 hours.

  a. Would you use a macrodrip or microdrip IV set?

  _____.

  b. Determine which IV set to use and then calculate the drops per minute (gtts/min) using one of the three methods.

2. Order: 3 liters of IV solutions for 24 hours: 2 liters of 5% D/½ NSS and 1 liter of D_5W.

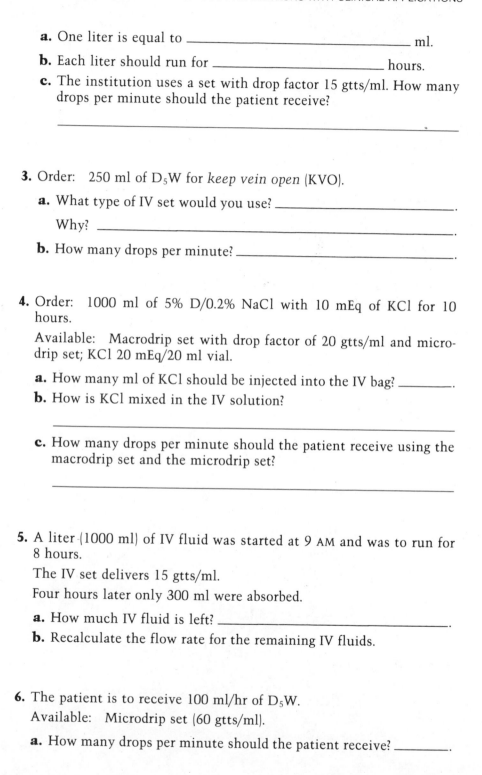

   a. One liter is equal to _____ ml.

   b. Each liter should run for _____ hours.

   c. The institution uses a set with drop factor 15 gtts/ml. How many drops per minute should the patient receive?

   _____

3. Order: 250 ml of D$_5$W for *keep vein open* (KVO).

   a. What type of IV set would you use? _____.

   Why? _____.

   b. How many drops per minute? _____.

4. Order: 1000 ml of 5% D/0.2% NaCl with 10 mEq of KCl for 10 hours.

   Available: Macrodrip set with drop factor of 20 gtts/ml and microdrip set; KCl 20 mEq/20 ml vial.

   a. How many ml of KCl should be injected into the IV bag? _____.

   b. How is KCl mixed in the IV solution?

   _____

   c. How many drops per minute should the patient receive using the macrodrip set and the microdrip set?

   _____

5. A liter (1000 ml) of IV fluid was started at 9 AM and was to run for 8 hours.

   The IV set delivers 15 gtts/ml.

   Four hours later only 300 ml were absorbed.

   a. How much IV fluid is left? _____.

   b. Recalculate the flow rate for the remaining IV fluids.

6. The patient is to receive 100 ml/hr of D$_5$W.

   Available: Microdrip set (60 gtts/ml).

   a. How many drops per minute should the patient receive? _____.

ANSWERS

1. a. Microdrip set, since the patient is to receive 83 ml/hr.

    b. Method I: (a) $\dfrac{1000}{12} = 83$ ml/hr;   (b) $\dfrac{83}{60} = 1.38$ ml/min;

              (c) 1.4 ml/min $\times$ 60 gtts/ml = 84 gtts/min

Using a microdrip set (60 gtts/ml), IV should run 84 gtts/min.

2. a. 1 liter = 1000 ml.

    b. Each liter should run for 8 hours.

    c. Method II: 1000 ÷ 8 = 125 ml/hr

$$\frac{125 \times \overset{1}{\cancel{15}}}{\underset{4}{\cancel{60}}} = \frac{125}{4} = 31\text{--}32 \text{ gtts/min}$$

Using a 15 gtts/ml drop set, IV should run 31–32 gtts/min.

3. a. Microdrip set with drop factor of 60 gtts/ml.

    b. Method III: $\dfrac{250 \times \overset{1}{\cancel{60}}}{24 \times \underset{1}{\cancel{60}}} = 10$ gtts/min

Using a microdrip set, IV should run 10 gtts/min. KVO usually means 24 hours.

4. a. 10 ml of KCl.

    b. Use a 10 ml syringe and withdraw 10 ml of KCl. Inject into the rubber port stopper of the IV bag.

    c. Microdrip set: 100 gtts/min.
        Macrodrip set: Drop factor of 20 gtts/ml.
                       34 gtts/min.

5. a. 700 ml of IV fluid is left and 4 hours are left.

    b. Recalculate using 700 ml and 4 hours to run.

      Method I: (a) $\dfrac{700}{4} = 175$ ml/hr;

                 (b) $\dfrac{175}{60} = 2.9$ ml/min;

                 (c) 2.9 $\times$ 15 = 44 gtts/min

6. a. 100 gtts/min.

      Method II: $\dfrac{100 \times \overset{1}{\cancel{60}} \text{ gtts/ml}}{\underset{1}{\cancel{60}} \text{ min}} = 100$ gtts/min

INTERMITTENT INTRAVENOUS ADMINISTRATION

Some IV medications are prescribed three to four times a day and are administered in a small volume of IV fluid (50 to 100 ml of D_5W or saline). The drug solution is usually delivered to the patient in 15 minutes to 1 hour. A separate tube for IV drugs, the secondary line, is inserted into a port (rubber stopper) of the IV connector on the continuous or primary IV line. This type of IV administration is called intermittent IV therapy.

Secondary IV Sets Without Controllers

Two sets available for administering IV drugs are (1) the calibrated cylinder (chamber) with tubing, such as the Buretrol, Volutrol, and Soluset; and (2) the secondary set, which is similar to a regular IV set except that the tubing is shorter. The secondary set is primarily used for infusing small volumes, 50, 100, 250 ml bags or bottles. The chamber of the Buretrol, Volutrol, and Soluset holds 150 ml of solution. Medication is injected into the chamber, then diluted with solution. These methods for administering IV drugs are referred to as IV piggyback (IVPB).

Normally drugs for IV infusion are diluted prior to infusion. Clinical agencies frequently have their own protocols for dilutions; if not, the drug circular should have infusion guidelines. If the information is not available, the hospital pharmacy should be contacted. Guidelines and protocols help in preventing drug and fluid incompatibility.

When using the Buretrol, 15 ml of IV solution should be added to flush the drug out of the IV line once the drug infusion is completed. Usually, drugs administered by Buretrol, Volutrol, or Soluset are prepared by the nurse.

Intermittent Infusion Adapters (Heparin Lock)

When continuous IV fluid infusion is unnecessary but intermittent drug therapy must be continued, an adapter can be attached to the IV catheter or needle to close the connection that was attached to the IV tubing. Adapters have ports (stoppers) where needles or IV tubing can be inserted as necessary to continue drug therapy. Therefore, less solution is needed to keep the vein open, thus preventing excessive fluid intake. The use of adapters can allow the patient more mobility and can be cost-effective because less IV tubing, IV solution, and regulating equipment are needed. This type of device is sometimes referred to as a heparin lock.

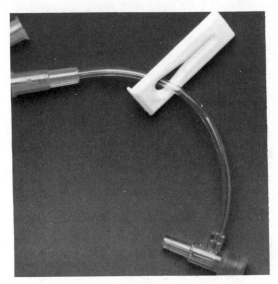

T-Port Set (IV adapter). Burron Medical, Inc., Bethlehem, PA.

IV catheters and needles with adapters are kept free from clotting by administering low doses of heparin after each drug infusion. In some institutions this is known as the SASH procedure. Before any drug is given, the IV tubing and adapter are flushed with 2 ml of saline solution, for the purpose of clearing the line of heparin solution and assessing for IV patency. After the drug is administered, a 2 ml saline flush is given, followed by a low dose of heparin.

The procedure stands for:

S = Solution (saline) flush (2 ml)
A = Administer drug into rubber stopper
S = Solution (saline) flush (2 ml)
H = Heparin 1:100 flush

Electronic Intravenous Regulators

Controllers and pumps are the two basic types of electronic intravenous regulators. Controllers work by the pressure that gravity exerts on the fluid in the IV container, bag, or bottle. They have an electronically controlled clamp that adjusts the flow by clamping and releasing the IV tubing. The controller's drop sensor on the drip chamber detects any

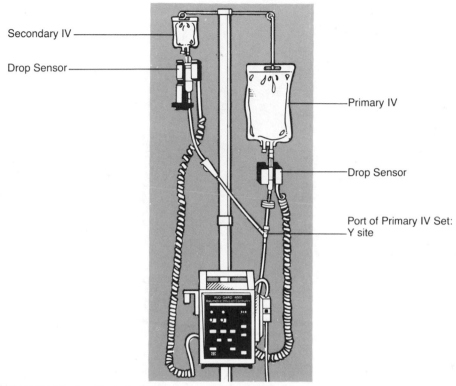

Secondary IV

Drop Sensor

Primary IV

Drop Sensor

Port of Primary IV Set: Y site

Volumetric Infusion Controller: Baxter-Travenol Laboratories, Deerfield, IL.

increase or decrease of drops, which automatically adjusts the clamp. Controllers are sensitive to any restrictions, such as infiltrations, and an alarm is sounded when the set rate cannot be maintained. Controllers are not accurate for volumes less than 5 ml/hr. To ensure the correct rate of infusion, the IV bag or bottle must be three feet above the IV site and the tubing must be free of occlusions.

There are two types of pumps, the IV regulator pump and the syringe pump. The IV pump will work on gravity but exerts positive pressure if there is any resistance. Pumps do not recognize infiltrations. The alarm will not sound until the pump has exerted its maximum pressure to overcome resistance. Syringe pumps are primarily used when a small volume of medication is given. Some syringe pumps can operate with syringes of various size, from tuberculin to 35 ml. Syringe pumps are primarily used in the neonatal and critical care units.

IV pumps are recommended for use with all central lines, such as arterial, femoral, and hyperalimentation. Controllers are used for peripheral lines, especially if fluid overload is a concern.

Another type of regulator that is inexpensive but not as accurate as the electronic devices is the Dial-A-Flow. The dial on the tubing is turned to the desired rate of IV flow per hour (ml/hr); it is primarily used for controlling large volumes of IV solutions.

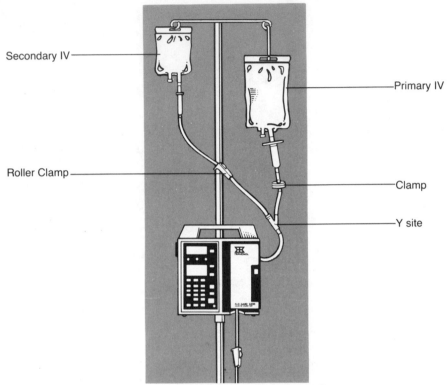

Volumetric Infusion Pump: Baxter-Travenol Laboratories, Deerfield, IL.

Flow Rates for Regulators. Determining the flow rates for electronic regulators depends on whether the type of flow control is volumetric or nonvolumetric. Volumetric regulators deliver a specific volume of fluid at a specific rate, measured in *ml/hr*. Nonvolumetric regulators are designed to infuse at a drop rate, *gtts/min*. Distinguishing between volumetric and nonvolumetric regulators involves checking the calibration on the machine display for ml/hr or gtts/min.

Calculating Flow Rates for IV Drugs

IV drug infusion rates depend upon (1) the drug dosing instruction, which indicates the amount of solution for dilution, and (2) the length of infusion time. The nurse must first calculate the drug dose from the physician's order, then calculate the flow rate.

I. Secondary sets, calibrated cylinders, and nonvolumetric regulators use *gtts/minute*. To find gtts/minute when administering IV drugs, use the *two-step method*.

1. $\dfrac{\text{Amount of solution}}{\text{Minutes to administer}} = \text{ml/min}$

2. ml/min $\times$ drops (gtts)/ml of IV set = gtts/min

II. Volumetric regulators use *ml/hr*. Use *one* of the following methods to calculate ml/hr.

a. ml/min × 60 minutes/hr = ml/hr

or

b. Amount of solution ÷ $\dfrac{\text{minutes to administer}}{\text{60 minutes/hr}}$ = ml/hr

EXAMPLES

Problems for calculating IV drug dosage and IV flow rate by *gtts/min* and *ml/hr* are given.

Problem 1: Order: Tagamet 200 mg, IV, q6h.

Drug available: cimetidine/Tagamet 300 mg/2 ml vial in aqueous solution.

Set and solution: Buretrol set with drop factor of 60 gtts/ml; 500 ml of D_5W.

Instruction: Dilute drug in 100 ml of D_5W and infuse in 20 minutes.

Drug Calculation:

$$\frac{D}{H} \times V =$$

$$\frac{200}{300} \times 2 = \frac{400}{300}$$

$$X = 1.3 \text{ ml of Tagamet}$$

H : V :: D : X
300 : 2 :: 200 : X

$$300\,X = 400 \qquad\qquad 1.3$$
$$X = \frac{400}{300} = 300\,\overline{)400.0}$$

$$X = 1.3 \text{ ml of Tagamet}$$

Flow Rate Calculation:

a. $\dfrac{\text{Amt of sol}}{\text{Min to adm}}$ = ml/min $\dfrac{100}{20}$ = 5 ml/min

b. ml/min × gtts/ml = gtts/min
    5   ×   60   = 300 gtts/min

Answer: Inject 1.3 ml of Tagamet into 100 ml of D_5W in the Buretrol chamber.

Regulate IV flow rate to 300 gtts/min.

It would be impossible to count 300 drops per minute. Instead of using the Buretrol, the nurse could use a secondary set having a larger drop factor or a regulator. If the Buretrol is the only available secondary IV set, then the 300 gtts/min should be approximated.

Problem 2: Order: Mandol 500 mg, IV, q6h.

Drug available: cefamandole/Mandol 2 g vial in powdered form. Add 6.6 ml of diluent = 8 ml of drug solution (2 g = 8 ml).

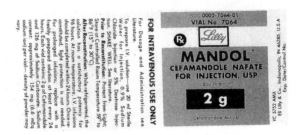

Set and solution: secondary set with 100 ml D$_5$W. Drop factor 15 gtts/ml.

Instruction: dilute in 100 ml of D$_5$W and infuse in 30 minutes.

Drug Calculation: (2.0 g = 2.000 mg)

$$\frac{D}{H} \times V =$$

$$\frac{500}{2000} \times 8 =$$

$$\frac{4000}{2000} = 2 \text{ ml of Mandol}$$

H	:	V	::	D	:	X
2000	:	8	::	500	:	X

2000 X = 4000

X = 2 ml of Mandol

Flow Rate Calculation:

a. $\dfrac{\text{Amt of sol}}{\text{Min to adm}} = \text{ml/min}$ $\dfrac{100}{30} = 3.3 \text{ ml/min}$

b. ml/min × gtts/ml = gtts/min
   3.3 × 15 = 49.5 or 50 gtts/min

Answer: Inject 2 ml of Mandol into the 100 ml D$_5$W bag.

Regulate IV flow rate at 50 gtts/min.

Problem 3: Order: ampicillin/Polycillin-N 1 g, IV, q6h.

Drug available:

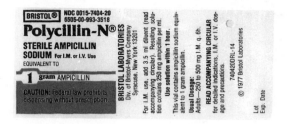

Add 4.5 ml of diluent, which equal 5 ml.

Set: use a volumetric pump.

Instruction: dilute in 50 ml of D_5W and infuse over 15 minutes.

Drug Calculation: Ampicillin 1 g = 5 ml of drug solution.

Volumetric Pump Rate: Amount of solution $\div \dfrac{\text{min to adm}}{60 \text{ min}} = \text{ml/hr}$

$$55 \text{ ml} \div \frac{15 \text{ min}}{60 \text{ min}} = 55 \times \frac{\overset{4}{\cancel{60}}}{\underset{1}{\cancel{15}}} = 220 \text{ ml/hr}$$

NOTE: Amount of solution is 50 ml of D_5W + 5 ml medication = 55 ml.

Answer: Rate on volumetric pump should be set at 220 ml/hr to deliver ampicillin 1 g in 15 minutes.

Problem 4: Order: albumin 25 g, IV.

Available: albumin 25 g in 50 ml.

Set: use a volumetric pump.

Instruction: administer over 25 minutes or 2 ml/minute.

Drug Calculation: Not applicable.

Volumetric Pump Rate:

$$2 \text{ ml/min} \times 60 \text{ min/hr} = 120 \text{ ml/hr}$$

or

$$50 \text{ ml} \div \frac{25 \text{ min}}{60 \text{ min}} = 50 \times \frac{60}{25} = \frac{3000}{25} = 120 \text{ ml/hr}$$

Answer: Volumetric rate should be set at 120 ml/hr.

Practice Problems

Calculate the fluid rate by using a calibrated cylinder (Buretrol) or secondary set and a volumetric pump.

1. Order: nafcillin/Nafcil 1 g, IV, q6h.

Drug available: nafcillin 2 g in powdered form in vial.

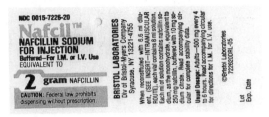

Set and solution: Buretrol set with drop factor of 60 gtts/ml; volumetric pump; 500 ml of D_5W.

Instruction: dilute drug in 75 ml of D_5W and infuse in 40 minutes.

Drug Calculation:

Flow Rate Calculation (gtts/min):
How many drops per minute should the patient receive using the Buretrol set?

_____

Volumetric Pump Rate (ml/hr):
With volumetric pump, how many ml/hr?

_____

2. Order: piperacillin 2.5 g, IV, q6h.

Drug available: piperacillin 4 g vial in powdered form. Add 7.8 ml of diluent to yield 10 ml of drug solution (4 g = 10 ml).

Set and solution: Buretrol set with drop factor of 60 gtts/ml; volumetric pump; 500 ml of D_5W.

Instruction: dilute drug in 100 ml of D_5W and infuse in 30 minutes.

Drug Calculation:

Flow Rate Calculation (gtts/min):
How many drops per minute should the patient receive using the Buretrol set?

_____

Volumetric Pump Rate (ml/hr):
With a volumetric pump, how many ml/hr?

_____

3. Order: methicillin/Staphcillin 1 g, IV, q6h.

Drug available: Staphcillin 4 g in powdered form in vial. Add 5.7 ml of diluent to yield 8 ml.

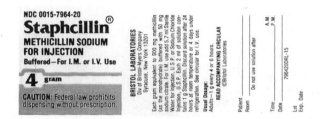

Set and solution: secondary set with drop factor 15 gtts/ml; 100 ml bag of D₅W; volumetric pump.

Instruction: dilute drug in 100 ml of D$_5$W and infuse in 40 minutes.

Drug Calculation:
Explain the procedure for diluting drug and adding to IV bag.

Flow Rate Calculation (gtts/min):
How many drops per minute should the patient receive using a secondary set?

_____

Volumetric Pump Rate (ml/hr):
With a volumetric pump, how many ml/hr?

_____

4. Order: Vibramycin 100 mg, IV, q12h.

   Drug available: doxycycline/Vibramycin 100 mg vial in powdered form. Add 10 ml of diluent.

   Set and solution: secondary set with drop factor 15 gtts/ml; 100 ml of D_5W; volumetric pump; nonvolumetric pump.

   Instruction: dilute 10 ml in 90 ml of D_5W and infuse in 60 minutes. Dilution should be 1 mg = 1 ml.

Drug Calculation:
Is the dilution ratio to mg per ml correct?

_____

Flow Rate Calculation (gtts/min):
What is the IV flow rate using a secondary set?

_____

Volumetric Pump Rate (ml/hr):
With a volumetric pump, how many ml/hr?

_____

Nonvolumetric Pump Rate (gtts/min):
With a nonvolumetric pump, how many gtts/min?

_____

ANSWERS

1. *Drug Calculation:*   Nafcillin 2 g = 8 ml; 1 g = 4 ml.

   Flow Rate Calculation: Total solution: 75 ml D_5W + 4 ml of drug solution = 79 ml.

   a. $\dfrac{79}{40} = 1.98$ ml/min   **b.** $1.98 \times 60 = 119$ gtts/min

   Volumetric Pump Rate:

   a. 1.98 ml/min $\times$ 60 min/hr = 119 ml/hr

   or

   b. 79 ml $\div \dfrac{40}{60} = 79 \times \dfrac{60}{40} = 79 \times \dfrac{3}{2} = \dfrac{237}{2} = 119$ ml/hr

Set volumetric rate at 119 ml/hr to deliver nafcillin 1 g in 40 minutes.

2. *Drug Calculation:*

$$\frac{D}{H} \times V = \frac{2.5}{4} \times 10 = 6.25 \text{ ml of piperacillin}$$

Flow Rate Calculation: Total solution: 100 ml D$_5$W + 6 ml of drug solution = 106 ml.

a. $\dfrac{106}{30} = 3.5$ ml/min

b. $3.5 \times 60 = 210$ gtts/min

Volumetric Pump Rate:

$$3.5 \text{ ml/min} \times 60 \text{ min/hr} = 210 \text{ ml/hr}$$

Set volumetric rate at 210 ml/hr to deliver piperacillin 2.5 g in 30 minutes.

3. *Drug Calculation:* Staphcillin 4 g = 8 ml. Withdraw 2 ml from vial to yield Staphcillin 1 g.

Flow Rate Calculation: Total solution: 100 ml D$_5$W + 2 ml of drug solution = 102 ml of IV solution.

a. $\dfrac{102}{40} = 2.55$ ml/min

b. $2.55 \times 15 = 38$ gtts/min

Inject 2 ml of Staphcillin into 100 ml of D$_5$W bag. Rotate bag.

Volumetric Pump Rate:

$$2.55 \text{ ml/min} \times 60 \text{ min/hr} = 153 \text{ ml/hr}$$

Set volumetric rate at 153 ml/hr to deliver Staphcillin 1 g in 40 minutes.

4. *Drug Calculation:* Mix 10 ml of diluent with Vibramycin 100 mg in vial.

Flow Rate Calculation: Expel 10 ml of IV solution. Inject 10 ml of drug solution in 90 ml of IV solution.

a. $\dfrac{100}{60} = 1.7$ ml/min

b. $1.7 \times 15 = 25.5$ or 26 gtts/min

Volumetric Pump Rate:

$$1.7 \text{ ml/min} \times 60 \text{ min/hr} = 102 \text{ ml/hr}$$

Set volumetric rate at 102 ml/hr to deliver Vibramycin 100 mg in 60 minutes.

Nonvolumetric Pump Rate:
Same as the flow rate calculation: gtts/minute (26 gtts/min).

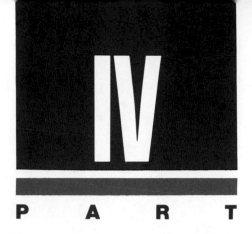

IV

P A R T

Calculations for Specialty Areas

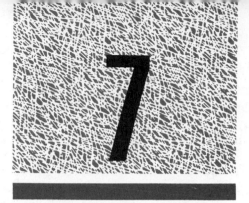

C H A P T E R

Pediatrics

Objectives

- Utilize the two primary methods in determining pediatric drug dosages.
- State the reason for checking pediatric dosages prior to administration.
- Describe the dosage inaccuracies that may occur with pediatric drug formulas.
- Identify the steps in determining body surface area from a pediatric nomogram.

Drug dosages for children differ greatly from those for adults because of physiological differences. Neonates and infants have immature kidney and liver function, which delays metabolism and elimination of many drugs. Also, drug absorption is altered as a result of slow gastric emptying time. Decreased gastric acid secretion in children under 3 years contributes to altered drug absorption. Neonates and infants have a lower concentration of plasma proteins, which can cause toxicity with drugs that are highly bound to proteins. They have less total body fat and more total body water. Therefore, lipid-soluble drugs require smaller doses with less fat present, and water-soluble drugs may need larger doses because of a greater percentage of body water. As children grow, the changes in fat, muscle, body water, and organ maturity can alter the pharmacokinetics of drugs. It is the nurse's responsibility to ensure that a safe drug dosage is given, and to closely monitor signs and symptoms of adverse reactions to drugs. The purpose of learning how to calculate pediatric drug doses is to ensure that the child receives the correct dose within the therapeutic range.

The two main methods in determining drug dosages for pediatric drug administration are body weight and body surface area. The first method uses a specific number of milligrams, micrograms, or units for each kilogram of body weight (mg/kg, mcg/kg, U/kg). Usually drug data for pediatric dosage (mg/kg) are supplied by manufacturers with a drug information insert. Body surface area/BSA (m^2) is the other method, which is considered more accurate than body weight. It takes into consideration the relationship between basal metabolic rate and body surface area, which correlates with blood volume, cardiac output, and organ growth and development. Although m^2 has primarily been used for antineoplastic agents, manufacturers are beginning to include body surface parameters (mg/m^2, mcg/m^2, U/m^2) with drug information.

If the manufacturer does not supply data for pediatric dosing, the child's dosage can be determined from the adult dose. The body surface area rule is currently used to derive the pediatric dose. The BSA rule is considered more accurate than previously used formulas such as Clark's, Young's, and Fried's rules. Drug calculations according to the BSA rule are safer than formulas that relied solely on the child's age or weight. Although the BSA rule has improved drug dosing for infants and children, calculation of drug doses for neonates and preterm infants using this method does not guarantee complete accuracy.

PEDIATRIC DRUG CALCULATIONS
Dosage per Kilogram Body Weight

The following information is needed to calculate this dose:

a. Physician's order with the name of the drug, the dosage, and the frequency.

b. The child's weight in kilograms.

$$1 \text{ kg} = 2.2 \text{ lb.}$$

c. The pediatric dosage as listed by the manufacturer or hospital formulary.

d. Information on how the drug is supplied.

EXAMPLES

Problem 1: **a.** Order: amoxicillin 60 mg, p.o., tid.

Child's weight: 12½ lb.

b. Change pounds to kilograms.

$$\frac{12.5}{2.2} = 5.7 \text{ kg}$$

c. Pediatric dosage for under 20 kg: 20-40 mg/kg/day in three equal doses.

Step 1:   Check dosing parameters by multiplying the child's weight by the minimum and maximum daily dose of the drug.

$$20 \text{ mg/kg/day} \times 5.7 \text{ kg} = 114 \text{ mg/day}$$

$$40 \text{ mg/kg/day} \times 5.7 \text{ kg} = 228 \text{ mg/day}$$

Step 2:   Multiply the dosage by the frequency to determine the daily dose.

The order for amoxicillin 60 mg, p.o., tid means that three doses will be given per day.

$$60 \text{ mg} \times 3 = 180 \text{ mg}$$

Because the daily dose of amoxicillin 180 mg falls within the recommended range, it is considered a safe dose.

d. Drug preparation: amoxicillin oral suspension 125 mg/ 5 ml.

Use either the basic formula $\frac{D}{H} \times V$, ratio and proportion, or fraction equation.

Basic formula

$$\frac{60 \text{ mg}}{125 \text{ mg}} \times 5 \text{ ml} = 2.4 \text{ ml}$$

Ratio and Proportion

$$125 \text{ mg} : 5 \text{ ml} = 60 \text{ mg} : X$$
$$125 X = 300$$
$$X = 2.4 \text{ ml}$$

Answer: Amoxicillin 60 mg, p.o. = 2.4 ml.

Problem 2:   **a.** Order: digoxin 40 mcg, IV, bid.

One-month-old infant weighs: 6 lb.

b. Change pounds to kilograms.

$$\frac{6}{2.2} = 2.72 \text{ kg}$$

c. Pediatric dosage for children 2 weeks to 2 years old: 25–50 mcg/kg.

Step 1:   Multiply the weight by the minimum and maximum daily dose.

25 mcg/kg/day × 2.72 kg = 68 mcg

50 mcg/kg/day × 2.72 kg = 136 mcg

Step 2:   Multiply the dose by the frequency.

40 mcg × 2 = 80 mcg

The dose is considered safe because it is within the therapeutic range for the infant's weight.

d. Drug preparation: digoxin 0.1 mg/ml.

Use your selected formula to calculate the dosage. For ease of calculation, change the units of drug from mg to mcg (digoxin 0.1 mg/ml = digoxin 100 mcg/ml).

$$\frac{D}{H} \times V = \frac{40 \text{ mcg}}{100 \text{ mcg}} \times 1 \text{ ml} = 0.4 \text{ ml}$$

100 mcg : 1 ml = 40 mcg : X

100 X = 40

X = 0.4 ml

Answer: Each dose of digoxin 40 mcg is 0.4 ml.

Dosage per Body Surface Area/BSA

The following information is needed to calculate this dosage:

a. Physician's order with name of drug, dosage, and time frame/frequency.

b. Child's height, weight in kilograms, and age.

c. Information on how the drug is supplied.

d. Pediatric dosage in m^2 as listed by manufacturer or hospital formulary.

e. Body surface area nomogram for children.

EXAMPLE

Problem 1:   **a.** Order: methotrexate 50 mg, IV, × 1.

b. Child's ht, wt, age: 134 cm, 32.5 kg, 9 yrs.

c. Pediatric dose: 25–75 mg/m²/wk.

d. Drug preparation: 2.5 mg/ml, 25 mg/ml.

e. Body surface area nomogram for children: The child's height (134 cm) and weight (32.5 kg) intersect at 1.11 m² (BSA). (See nomogram, p. 138.)

Step 1: Multiply the BSA, 1.11 m², by the minimum and maximum dose. (Substitute BSA for weight.)

$$25 \text{ mg/m}^2 \times 1.1 \text{ m}^2 = 28.0 \text{ mg}$$

$$75 \text{ mg/m}^2 \times 1.1 \text{ m}^2 = 83.0 \text{ mg}$$

This dose is considered safe because it is within the therapeutic range for the child's body surface area.

f. Calculate drug dose: To determine the amount of drug to be administered, either formula can be used.

$$\frac{D}{H} \times V = \frac{50 \text{ mg}}{25 \text{ mg}} \times 1 \text{ ml} = 2 \text{ ml} \qquad \begin{array}{l} 25 \text{ mg} : 1 \text{ ml} = 50 \text{ mg} : X \\ 25 \text{ X} = 50 \\ X = 2 \text{ ml} \end{array}$$

Answer: Methotrexate 50 mg = 2 ml.

Practice Problems

With the following dosage problems for oral, IM, and IV administration, determine if the ordered dose is safe and how much of the drug should be given.

1. Treatment for a child with seizures.
   Order: Dilantin 40 mg, p.o., bid.
   Child's weight: 6.7 kg.
   Pediatric dose: 5–7 mg/kg/day.
   Drug available: Dilantin 30 mg/5 ml, suspension.

_____

2. Treatment for a child with a urinary tract infection.
   Order: Gantrisin 1.5 g, p.o., qid.
   Child's weight: 30.4 kg.
   Pediatric dose: 150–200 mg/kg/day.
   Drug available: Gantrisin 500 mg tablets.

_____

3. Child with cystic fibrosis exposed to influenza A.
   Order: Symmetrel 25 mg, p.o., tid.

Child's weight: 14 kg.
Pediatric dose: 4–8 mg/kg/day.
Drug available: Symmetrel 50 mg/5 ml.

---

4. Child with seizures.
   Order: phenobarbital 25 mg, p.o., bid.
   Child's weight: 7.2 kg.
   Pediatric dose: 5–7 mg/kg/day.
   Drug available: phenobarbital 20 mg/5 ml.

---

5. Child with pain.
   Order: codeine 7.5 mg, p.o., q4h, PRN × 6 doses/day.
   Child's height and weight: 43 inches, 50 lb.
   Pediatric dose: 100 mg/m^2/day.
   Drug available: codeine 15 mg tablets.

---

6. Child with cancer.
   Order: methotrexate 50 mg, IM, q weekly.
   Child's height and weight: 56 inches, 100 lb.
   Pediatric dose: 25–75 mg/m^2/wk
   Drug available: methotrexate 2.5 mg/ml; 25 mg/ml; 100 mg/ml.

---

7. Child has strep throat.
   Order: Bicillin C-R, 1,000,000 U, IM, stat.
   Child's weight: 44 lb.
   Pediatric dose: 30–60 lb: 900,000–1,200,000 U daily.
   Drug available: Bicillin C-R 1,200,000 U/2 ml.

---

8. Child is receiving preoperative medication.
   Order: hydroxyzine/Vistaril 25 mg, IM.
   Child's height and weight: 47 inches, 45 lb.
   Pediatric dose: 30 mg/m^2.
   Drug available: Vistaril 25 mg/ml.

---

9. Child has nausea post surgery.
   Order: Phenergan 20 mg, IM, q6h.
   Child's weight: 45 kg.

Pediatric dose: 0.25–0.5 mg/kg/dose, repeat 4–6 hr.
Drug available: Phenergan 25 mg/ml.

---

10. Child has 30% second-degree burns.
Order: morphine 2–3 mg, IM, q4h, PRN.
Child's weight and age: 15 kg, 3 years old.
Pediatric dose: 0.1–0.2 mg/kg/dose.
Drug available: morphine 10 mg/ml.

---

11. Child has pneumonia.
Order: ampicillin 500 mg, IV q6h.
Child's weight: 5.6 kg.
Pediatric dose: 300 mg/kg/day.
Drug available: ampicillin 250 mg/ml.

---

12. Child with head trauma.
Order: Decadron 2 mg, IV, q6h.
Child's weight and age: 10.1 kg, 16 months.
Pediatric dose: 0.4 mg/kg/day in divided doses.
Drug available: Decadron 10 mg/ml.

---

13. Child has sepsis.
Order: gentamicin 10 mg, IV, q8h.
Child's height, weight, age: 21 inches, 4 kg, 1 month.
Pediatric dose: > 7 days old: 5–7.5 mg/kg/day, 3–4 divided doses.
Drug available: gentamicin 10 mg/ml.

---

14. Child with cancer.
Order: Adriamycin 12 mg, IV, qd.
Child's height, weight, age: 44 inches, 18 kg, 5 years old.
Pediatric dose: 15–30 mg/m^2/day
Drug available: Adriamycin 50 mg/25 ml.

---

15. Child with infection.
Order: penicillin G 300,000 U, IV, q4h.
Child's weight and age: 9 kg, 18 months old.
Pediatric dose: 25,000–400,000 U/kg/day in 4–6 divided doses.

Drug available: penicillin G 1,000,000 U/5 ml.

ANSWERS

1. Dosage parameters: 5 mg/kg/day × 6.7 kg = 33.5 mg/day

7 mg/kg/day × 6.7 kg = 46.9 (47) mg/day

Dose frequency: 40 mg × 2 = 80 mg

Dosage exceeds the therapeutic range. Dosage is *not* safe.

2. Dosage parameters: 150 mg/kg/day × 30.4 = 4560 mg or 4.5 g

200 mg/kg/day × 30.4 = 6080 mg or 6.1 g

Dose frequency: 1.5 g × 4 = 6.0 g or 6000 mg

Dosage is safe.

$$\frac{D}{H} = \frac{1500}{500} \text{ mg} = 3 \text{ tablets per dose}$$

3. Dosage parameters: 4 mg/kg/day × 14 kg = 56 mg/day

8 mg/kg/day × 14 kg = 112 mg/day

Dose frequency: 25 mg × 3 = 75 mg

Dosage is safe.

$$\frac{D}{H} \times V = \frac{25 \text{ mg}}{50 \text{ mg}} \times 5 \text{ ml} = 2.5 \text{ ml per dose}$$

4. Dosage parameters: 5 mg/kg/day × 7.2 kg = 36 mg/day

7 mg/kg/day × 7.2 kg = 50.4 mg/day

Dose frequency: 25 mg × 2 = 50 mg

Dosage is safe.

$$\frac{D}{H} \times V = \frac{25 \text{ mg}}{20 \text{ mg}} \times 5 \text{ ml} = 6.25 \text{ ml per dose}$$

5. Height and weight intersect at 0.84 m²

Dosage parameters: 100 mg/0.84 m²/day = 84 mg/day

Dose frequency: 84 mg/day ÷ 6 = 14 mg/dose

Dosage is safe.

$$\frac{D}{H} \times V = \frac{7.5}{15} \times 1 = 0.50 \text{ or } \frac{1}{2} \text{ tablet}$$

½ tablet q4h, PRN

6. Height and weight intersect at 1.38 m²

Dosage parameters: 25 mg/m²/wk $\times$ 1.38 m² = 34.5 mg/wk

75 mg/m²/wk $\times$ 1.38 m² = 103.5 mg/wk

Dose frequency: 50 mg/wk, IM

Dosage is safe.

$$\frac{D}{H} \times V = \frac{50}{100} \text{ mg} \times 1 = 0.5 \text{ ml}$$

7. Dosage parameters:

Child's weight is 44 pounds. It falls in the 30–60 pounds of the pediatric dose range.

Dose frequency:

Stat dose of 1,000,000 U. It falls within the pediatric dose range.

Dosage is safe.

$$\frac{D}{H} \times V = \frac{1,000,000}{1,200,000} \text{ U} \times 2 = 1.6 \text{ ml}$$

8. Height and weight intersect at 0.82 m²

Dosage parameters: 30 mg/m² $\times$ 0.82 m² = 24.6 mg or 25 mg

Dose frequency: 25 mg, IM

Dosage is safe.

$$\frac{D}{H} \times V = \frac{25}{25} \text{ mg} \times 1 = 1.0 \text{ ml}$$

9. Dosage parameters: 0.25/kg/dose $\times$ 45 kg = 11.25 mg/dose

0.5/kg/dose $\times$ 45 kg = 22.5 mg/dose

Dose frequency: 20 mg IM per dose

Dosage is safe.

$$\frac{D}{H} \times V = \frac{20}{25} \text{ mg} \times 1 = 0.8 \text{ ml}$$

10. Dosage parameters: 0.1 mg/kg $\times$ 15 kg = 1.5 mg per dose

0.2 mg/kg $\times$ 15 kg = 3 mg per dose

Dose frequency: 2–3 mg IM per dose

Dosage is safe.

$$\frac{D}{H} \times V = \frac{2 \text{ mg}}{10 \text{ mg}} \times 1 = 0.2 \text{ ml} \qquad \frac{3 \text{ mg}}{10 \text{ mg}} \times 1 = 0.3 \text{ ml}$$

11. Dosage parameters: 300 mg $\times$ 5.6 kg = 1680 mg/day

    Dose frequency: 1680 mg $\div$ 4 doses = 420 mg per dose

    Dose exceeds therapeutic range of 300 mg per dose. Dosage is *not* safe.

12. Dosage parameters: 0.4 mg/kg/day $\times$ 10.1 kg = 4 mg/day

    Dose frequency:

    $$2 \text{ mg} \times 4 \text{ times/day} = 8 \text{ mg per day}$$

    or

    $$4 \text{ mg} \div 4 \text{ doses} = 1 \text{ mg per dose}$$

    Dose exceeds therapeutic range of 1 mg per dose. Dosage is *not* safe.

13. Dosage parameters: 5 mg/kg/day $\times$ 4 kg = 20 mg/day

    7.5 mg/kg/day $\times$ 4 kg = 30 mg/day

    Dose frequency: 10 mg $\times$ 3 times/day = 30 mg

    Dosage is safe.

    $$\frac{D}{H} \times V = \frac{10}{10} \times 1 = 1 \text{ ml}$$

14. Height and weight intersect at 0.74 m^2

    Dosage parameters: 15 mg/m^2/day $\times$ 0.74 = 11.1 mg

    30 mg/m^2/day $\times$ 0.74 = 22.2 mg

    Dose frequency: 12 mg IV per day

    Dosage is safe.

    $$\frac{D}{H} \times V = \frac{12}{50} \times 25 \text{ ml} = 6 \text{ ml}$$

15. Dosage parameters:

    $$25,000 \text{ U/kg/day} \times 9 \text{ kg} = 225,000 \text{ U/day}$$
    $$400,000 \text{ U/kg/day} \times 9 \text{ kg} = 3,600,000 \text{ U/day}$$

    Dose frequency:

    $$300,000 \text{ U} \times 6 \text{ doses} = 1,800,000 \text{ U/daily}$$

    Dosage is safe.

    $$\frac{D}{H} \times V = \frac{300,000}{1,000,000} \text{ U} \times 5 \text{ ml} = 1.5 \text{ ml}$$

PEDIATRIC DOSAGE FROM ADULT DOSAGE
Body Surface Area Rule

The following information is needed to calculate the pediatric dosage using the BSA rule:

a. Physician's order with the name of the drug, the dosage, and the time frame/frequency.

b. The child's height and weight in kilograms.

c. A body surface area nomogram for children.

d. The adult drug dosage.

e. The formula for the body surface area rule:

$$\frac{\text{Surface area } (m^2)}{1.73 \ m^2} \times \text{Adult dose} = \text{Child's dose}$$

EXAMPLE

Problem 1: **a.** Erythromycin 80 mg, p.o., qid.

b. Child's height is 34 inches, and weight is 28.5 lb.
NOTE: Height and weight do not have to be converted to the metric system.

c. Height (34 inches) and weight (28.5 lb) intersect the nomogram at 0.57 m². See BSA nomogram scale, p. 138.

d. The adult drug dosage is 1000 mg/24 hr.

e. Body surface area rule:

$$\frac{\text{Surface area } (m^2)}{1.73 \ m^2} \times \text{Adult dose} =$$

$$\frac{0.57 \ m^2}{1.73 \ m^2} \times 1000 =$$

$$0.33 \times 1000 = 330 \ mg/24 \ hr$$

Dose frequency:

$$330 \ mg \div 4 \ doses = 82.5$$

or

$$80 \ mg \ per \ dose$$

Dosage is safe.

$$80 \ mg \times 4 \ times \ a \ day = 320 \ mg/day$$

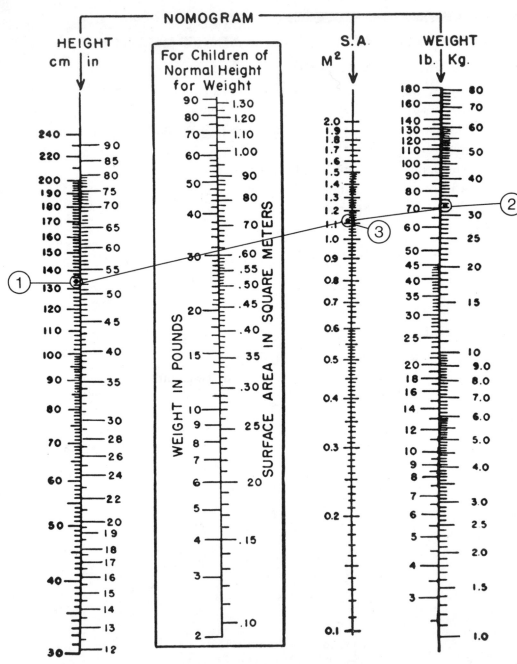

West Nomogram: Dosages for Infants and Children.

Directions: (1) Find height; (2) find weight; (3) draw a straight line from 1 and 2, and where the line intersects on the SA column is the body surface area (m²).

(From Behrman, R.E., and Vaughan, V.C.: Nelson Textbook of Pediatrics. Philadelphia, W.B. Saunders Co., 1987.)

Age Rules

Fried's rule and Young's rule are two methods in determining pediatric drug doses based on the child's age. Fried's rule is primarily used for children under 1 year of age, whereas Young's rule is for children between 2 and 12 years. In current practice these rules are infrequently used. Since the maturational development of infants and children is variable, age cannot be an accurate basis for drug dosing.

Fried's Rule:

$$\frac{\text{age in months}}{150} \times \text{adult dose} = \text{infant's dose}$$

Young's Rule:

$$\frac{\text{child's age in years}}{\text{age in years} + 12} \times \text{adult dose} = \text{child's dose}$$

Body Weight Rule

Clark's rule is another method to derive a pediatric dosage based upon the child's weight in pounds and the average adult weight of 150 lb. Population studies have shown an increase in the average weight of adults, therefore making 150 lb an inaccurate constant in the rule. Using the fixed constant in Clark's rule can lead to the underdosing of infants. Clark's rule is being phased out as a method for determining drug dosage in children.

Clark's Rule:

$$\frac{\text{child's wt in lb}}{150 \text{ lb}} \times \text{adult dose} = \text{child's dose}$$

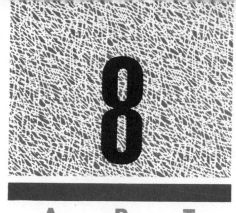

8

C H A P T E R

Critical Care

Objectives

- Calculate the prescribed concentration of a drug in solution.
- Identify the units of measure designated for the amount of drug in solution.
- Describe the differences in infusion rates for concentration and volume.
- Calculate the concentration of drug per unit time for a specific body weight.
- Recognize the variables needed for the basic fractional equation.
- Describe how the titration factor is used when infusion rates are changed.
- Recognize the methods of determining the total amount of drug infused over time.

Medication administration is becoming more individualized in the specialty areas. Many times it is necessary to calculate the patient's dose in micrograms per kilogram of body weight per minute or in units per hour. As the patient's condition changes, medications may be added or discontinued, which necessitates calculating the total amount of drug administered over a short period of time. Administration of potent drugs, in milligrams, micrograms, or units per body weight or unit time, requires extreme accuracy in calculations. Drug manufacturers provide dosage administration charts for quick reference to initiate drug treatment. Most charts use ranges of weight or rates that prevent individualization of drug doses. Basic knowledge of calculations used to determine administration of individualized dosage can validate the accuracy of the dosage chosen from an administration chart.

Physicians determine the amount of drug to be mixed in the infusate (solution) and designate infusion rates or the dosage per kilogram of body weight per unit time. Some institutions have their own guidelines for preparation of medication in the critical care areas, but the administration and calculation of the actual dose is a nursing function.

The mathematical skills needed to work problems in this chapter include the knowledge of proper and improper fractions, cancellation of units, ratio and proportion, and conversion to the metric system.

CALCULATING AMOUNT OF DRUG OR CONCENTRATION OF A SOLUTION

The first step for administering medication is to determine the concentration of the solution, which is the amount of drug in each milliliter of solution. This is written as units/milliliter, milligrams/milliliter, or micrograms/milliliter and must be calculated for each problem.

Calculating Units/Milliliter

EXAMPLE

Problem: Infuse heparin 5000 units in D_5W 250 ml at 30 ml/hr.

What will be the concentration of heparin in each ml of D_5W?

METHOD:	units/ml

Set up a ratio/proportion. Solve for X.	5000 units : 250 ml = X units : ml

$$250 X = 5000$$
$$X = 20 \text{ units}$$

Answer: The D₅W with heparin will have a concentration of *20 units/ml* of solution.

Calculating Milligrams/Milliliter

EXAMPLE

Problem: Infuse lidocaine 2 g in 500 ml D₅W at 2 mg/minute. What will be the concentration of lidocaine in each ml of D₅W?

| METHOD: | mg/ml |

| Convert grams to milligrams. Set up a ratio/proportion and solve for X. |

$$2 \text{ g} = 2000 \text{ mg}$$
$$2000 \text{ mg} : 500 \text{ ml} = X \text{ mg} : \text{ml}$$

$$500 \text{ X} = 2000$$
$$X = 4 \text{ mg}$$

Answer: The D₅W with lidocaine has a concentration of *4 mg/ml* of solution.

Calculating Micrograms/Milliliter

EXAMPLE

Problem: Infuse Isuprel 2 mg in 500 ml D₅W at 5 mcg/minute. What is the concentration of Isuprel in each ml of D₅W?

| METHOD: | mcg/ml |

| Convert milligrams to micrograms. Set up a ratio/proportion and solve for X. |

$$2 \text{ mg} = 2000 \text{ mcg}$$
$$2000 \text{ mcg} : 500 \text{ ml} = X \text{ mcg} : \text{ml}$$

$$500 \text{ X} = 2000$$
$$X = 4 \text{ mcg}$$

Answer: The D₅W with Isuprel will have a concentration of *4 mcg/ml* of solution.

Practice Problems

1. Infuse heparin 10,000 units in 250 ml D₅W at 30 ml/hr.

2. Infuse Aminophyllin 250 mg in 500 ml D$_5$W at 50 ml/hr.

_____

3. Order: regular insulin 100 units in 500 ml NS at 30 ml/hr.

_____

4. Order: lidocaine 1 g in 1000 ml D$_5$W at 30 ml/hr.

_____

5. Order: norepinephrine 4 mg in 500 ml D$_5$W at 15 ml/hr.

_____

6. Order: Dobutrex 500 mg in 250 ml D$_5$W at 10 ml/hr.

_____

7. Infuse Intropin 400 mg in 250 ml D$_5$W at 20 ml/hr.

_____

8. Infuse Isuprel 2 mg in 250 ml D$_5$W at 10 ml/hr.

_____

9. Order: streptokinase 750,000 units in 50 ml D$_5$W over 30 minutes.

_____

10. Order: nitroprusside 50 mg in 500 ml D$_5$W at 50 mcg/minute.

_____

ANSWERS

1. 10,000 units : 250 ml : : X units : ml
$$250 X = 10,000$$
$$X = 40 \text{ units}$$
The concentration of solution is 40 units/ml.

2. 250 mg : 500 ml : : X mg : ml
$$500 X = 250$$
$$X = 0.5 \text{ mg}$$
The concentration of solution is 0.5 mg/ml.

3. 100 units : 500 ml : : X units : ml
$$500 X = 100$$
$$X = 0.2 \text{ units}$$
The concentration of solution is 0.2 units/ml.

4.
$$1 \text{ g} = 1000 \text{ mg}$$
1000 mg : 1000 ml : : X mg : ml
$$1000 X = 1000$$
$$X = 1 \text{ mg}$$
The concentration of solution is 1 mg/ml.

5.
$$4 \text{ mg} = 4000 \text{ mcg}$$
4000 mcg : 500 ml : : X mcg : ml
$$500 X = 4000$$
$$X = 8 \text{ mcg}$$
The concentration of solution is 8 mcg/ml.

6. 500 mg : 250 ml : : X mcg : ml

      250 X = 500

          X = 2 mg

The concentration of solution is 2 mg/ml.

7. 400 mg : 250 ml : : X mg : ml

      250 X = 400

          X = 1.6 mg

The concentration of solution is 1.6 mg/ml.

8.   2 mg = 2000 mcg

  2000 mcg : 250 ml : : X mcg : ml

      250 X = 2000

          X = 8 mcg

The concentration of solution is 8 mcg/ml.

9. 750,000 units : 50 ml : : X units : ml

      50 X = 750,000

          X = 15,000 units

The concentration of solution is 15,000 units/ml.

10.   50 mg = 50,000 mcg

  50,000 mcg : 500 ml : : X mcg : ml

      500 X = 50,000

          X = 100 mcg

The concentration of solution is 100 mcg/ml.

CALCULATING INFUSION RATE FOR CONCENTRATION AND VOLUME PER UNIT TIME

The second step for administering medication is to calculate the *infusion rate* of drug per *unit time*. Infusion rate can mean two things, the rate of volume (ml) given or the rate of concentration (units, mg, mcg) administered. Infusion rates are usually part of the physician's order and may be stated in concentration or volume. The administration of potent drugs may be ordered by concentration per unit time. Unit time means per hour or per minute.

The widespread use of microdrip IV administration sets for the delivery of potent drugs and the use of volumetric infusion pumps, which are calibrated in ml/hr, limit the need for calculating infusion rates in drops per minute. As noted in Chapter 6, when using the microdrop administration set, the milliliter/hour rate corresponds to the drop rate/minute. Currently, the concentration per volume per unit time is the most accurate and safest method of drug administration. Potent drugs should always be administered with volumetric infusion pumps and in a closely monitored environment.

Concentration and Volume per Hour and Minute with a Drug in Units

EXAMPLE

Problem: Infuse heparin 5000 units in D_5W 250 ml at 30 ml/hr.

Concentration of solution is 20 units/ml. (See units/ml, page 142. Also note that volume/hr is given.)

How many milliliters will infuse per minute?

Find volume per minute.

METHOD:	ml/min

Set up a ratio/proportion. Use volume/hour, 30 ml/hr, or 30 ml/60 min as the known variable.	30 ml : 60 min : : X ml : min 60 X = 30 X = 0.5 ml

Answer: The infusion rate for volume per minute is *0.5 ml/min* and the hourly rate is *30 ml/hr.*

What is the concentration per minute and hour?

Find concentration per minute.

METHOD:	units/min

Multiply the concentration of solution by the volume per minute.	20 units/ml × 0.5 ml/min = 10 units/min

Find concentration per hour.

METHOD:	units/hr

Multiply the volume per minute by 60 min/hr.	10 units/min × 60 min/hr = 600 units/hr

Answer: The concentration per minute of heparin is *10 units/min* and the concentration per hour is *600 units/hr.*

Concentration and Volume per Hour and Minute with a Drug in Milligrams

EXAMPLE

Problem: Infuse lidocaine 2 g in D_5W 500 ml at 2 mg/minute.

Concentration of solution is 4 mg/ml. (See mg/ml, page 143. Note, also, concentration/min is given.)

How many milligrams will be infused per hour?

Find concentration per hour.

METHOD: mg/hr

Find the concentration/minute. Multiply concentration/min × 60 min/hr.	lidocaine 2 mg/min 2 mg/min × 60 min = 120 mg/hr

Answer: The amount of lidocaine infused per hour is *120 mg/hr.*

How many milliliters of lidocaine will infuse in one hour?

Find volume per hour.

METHOD: ml/hr

Calculate concentration of solution (see mg/ml, page 143). Divide the concentration/hr by the concentration of solution.	lidocaine 4 mg/ml $\dfrac{120 \text{ mg/hr}}{4 \text{ mg/ml}}$ = 30 ml/hr

Answer: The infusion rate in milliliters for lidocaine 2 mg/min is *30 ml/hr.*

How many milliliters of lidocaine will infuse in one minute?

Find volume per minute.

METHOD: ml/min

Divide the concentration/min by the concentration of solution.	$\dfrac{2 \text{ mg/min}}{4 \text{ mg/ml}}$ = 0.5 ml/min

Answer: The infusion rate for lidocaine 2 mg/min is *0.5 ml/min.*

Concentration and Volume per Minute and Hour with a Drug in Micrograms

EXAMPLE

Problem: Infuse Isuprel 2 mg in D₅W 500 ml at 5 mcg/minute.

Concentration of solution is 4 mcg/ml. (See mcg/ml, page 143. Note, also, concentration/min is given.)

How many micrograms will infuse in one hour?

Find concentration per hour.

METHOD:	**mcg/hr**

Find the concentration/minute. Multiply concentration/min × 60 min/hr.	Isuprel 5 mcg/min 5 mcg/min × 60 min/hr = 300 mcg/hr

Answer: The concentration of Isuprel infused per hour is *300 mcg/hr.*

How many milliliters of Isuprel will infuse in one hour?

Find volume per hour.

METHOD:	**ml/hr**

Calculate concentration of solution (see mcg/ml, p. 143). Divide the concentration/hr by the concentration of solution.	Isuprel 4 mcg/ml $\frac{300 \text{ mcg/hr}}{4 \text{ mcg/ml}}$ = 75 ml/hr

Answer: The infusion rate for Isuprel 5 mcg/min is *75 ml/hr.*

How many milliliters of Isuprel should infuse in one minute?

Find volume per minute.

METHOD:	**ml/min**

Divide concentration/min by concentration of solution.	$\frac{5 \text{ mcg/min}}{4 \text{ mcg/ml}}$ = 1.25 ml/min

Answer: The infusion rate for Isuprel 5 mcg/min is *1.25 ml/min.*

Practice Problems

Use the examples to find the following:

- Concentration of the solution
- Infusion rates per unit time

    a. volume/minute
    b. volume/hour
    c. concentration/minute
    d. concentration/hour

1. Order: heparin 1000 units in D_5W 500 ml at 50 ml/hr.

_____

2. Order: nitroprusside 100 mg in D_5W 500 ml at 60 ml/hr.

_____

3. Order: nitroprusside 25 mg in D_5W 250 ml at 50 mcg/min.

_____

4. Order: dopamine 800 mg in D_5W 500 ml at 400 mcg/min.

_____

5. Order: norepinephrine 2 mg in D_5W 250 ml at 45 ml/hr.

_____

6. Order: dobutamine 1000 mg in D_5W 500 ml at 12 ml/hr.

_____

7. Order: dobutamine 250 mg in D_5W 250 ml at 10 ml/hr.

_____

8. Order: lidocaine 2 g in D_5W 500 ml at 4 mg/min.

_____

9. Order: dopamine 400 mg in D_5W 250 ml at 60 ml/hr.

_____

10. Order: isoproterenol 4 mg in D_5W 500 ml at 65 ml/hr.

ANSWERS

1. *Concentration of solution*

    1000 units : 500 ml = X units : ml
            500 X = 1000   concentration of solution
               X = 2 units   2 units/ml

Infusion rates

a. Volume/min

50 ml : 60 min : : X ml : min
60 X = 50
X = 0.833 ml or 0.83 ml
0.83 ml/min

b. Volume/hr

50 ml/hr

c. Concentration/min

2 units/ml × 0.83 ml/min = 1.66 units/min

d. Concentration/hr

1.66 units/min × 60 min/hr = 99.6 units/hr
or 100 units/hr

2. *Concentration of solution*

100 mg : 500 ml : : X mg : ml
500 X = 100   concentration of solution
X = 0.2 mg   0.2 mg/ml

Infusion rates

a. Volume/min

60 ml : 60 min : : X ml : min
60 X = 60
X = 1 ml
1 ml/min

b. Volume/hr

60 ml/hr

c. Concentration/min

0.2 mg/ml × 1 ml/min = 0.2 mg/min

d. Concentration/hr

0.2 mg/min × 60 min/hr = 12 mg/hr

3. *Concentration of solution*

25 mg = 25,000 mcg
25,000 mcg : 250 ml : : X mcg : ml
250 X = 25,000   concentration of solution
X = 100 mcg   100 mcg/ml

Infusion rates

a. Volume/min

$$\frac{50 \text{ mcg/min}}{100 \text{ mcg/ml}} = 0.5 \text{ ml/min}$$

b. Volume/hr

0.5 ml/min × 60 min/hr
　　= 30 ml/hr

c. Concentration/min

50 mcg/min

d. Concentration/hr

50 mcg/min × 60 min/hr
　　= 3000 mcg/hr

4. *Concentration of solution*

　　　　　800 mg = 800,000 mcg
800,000 mcg : 500 ml : : X mcg : ml
　　　　500 X = 800,000　　　　　concentration of solution
　　　　　　X = 1600 mcg　　　　　1600 mcg/ml

Infusion rates

a. Volume/min

$$\frac{400 \text{ mcg/min}}{1600 \text{ mcg/ml}} = 0.25 \text{ ml/min}$$

b. Volume/hr

0.25 ml/min × 60 min/hr
　　= 15 ml/hr

c. Concentration/min

400 mcg/min

d. Concentration/hr

400 mcg/min × 60 min/hr
　　= 24,000 mcg/hr

5. *Concentration of solution*

　　　　　2 mg = 2000 mcg
2000 mcg : 250 ml : : X mcg : ml
　　　　250 X = 2000　　　　　concentration of solution
　　　　　　X = 8 mcg　　　　　8 mcg/ml

Infusion rates

a. Volume/min

$$45 \text{ ml} : 60 \text{ min} : : X \text{ ml} : \text{min}$$
$$60 X = 45$$
$$X = 0.75 \text{ ml/min}$$

b. Volume/hr

45 ml/hr

c. Concentration/min

$$8 \text{ mcg/ml} \times 0.75 \text{ ml/min} = 6 \text{ mcg/min}$$

d. Concentration/hr

$$6 \text{ mcg/min} \times 60 \text{ min/hr} = 360 \text{ mcg/hr}$$

6. *Concentration of solution*

$$1000 \text{ mg} = 1,000,000 \text{ mcg}$$
$$1,000,000 \text{ mcg} : 500 \text{ ml} : : X \text{ mcg} : \text{ml}$$
$$500 X = 1,000,000 \qquad \text{concentration of solution}$$
$$X = 2000 \text{ mcg} \qquad\qquad 2000 \text{ mcg/ml}$$

Infusion rates

a. Volume/min

$$12 \text{ ml} : 60 \text{ min} : : X \text{ ml} : \text{min}$$
$$60 X = 12$$
$$X = 0.2 \text{ ml}$$
$$0.2 \text{ ml/min}$$

b. Volume/hr

12 ml/hr

c. Concentration/min

$$2000 \text{ mcg/ml} \times 0.2 \text{ ml/min}$$
$$= 400 \text{ mcg/min}$$

d. Concentration/hr

$$400 \text{ mcg/min} \times 60 \text{ min/hr}$$
$$24,000 \text{ mcg/hr}$$

7. *Concentration of solution*

$$250 \text{ mg} = 250,000 \text{ mcg}$$
$$250,000 \text{ mcg} : 250 \text{ ml} : : X \text{ mcg} : \text{ml}$$
$$250 X = 250,000 \qquad \text{concentration of solution}$$
$$X = 1000 \text{ mcg} \qquad\qquad 1000 \text{ mcg/ml}$$

Infusion rates

a. Volume/min

$$10 \text{ ml} : 60 \text{ min} : : X \text{ ml} : 1 \text{ min}$$
$$60 \text{ X} = 10 \text{ ml}$$
$$X = 0.1666 \text{ ml or } 0.167 \text{ ml}$$
$$0.167 \text{ ml/min}$$

b. Volume/hr

10 ml/hr

c. Concentration/min

$$1000 \text{ mcg/ml} \times 0.167 \text{ ml/min}$$
$$= 167 \text{ mcg/min}$$

d. Concentration/hr

167 mcg/min $\times$ 60 min/hr = 10,020 mcg/hr or 10,000 mcg/hr

8. *Concentration of solution*

$$2 \text{ g} = 2000 \text{ mg}$$
$$2000 \text{ mg} : 500 \text{ ml} : : X \text{ mg} : \text{ml}$$
$$500 \text{ X} = 2000$$
$$X = 4 \text{ mg}$$

concentration of solution
4 mg/ml

Infusion rates

a. Volume/min

$$\frac{4 \text{ mg/ml}}{4 \text{ mg/min}} = 1 \text{ ml/min}$$

b. Volume/hr

1 ml/min $\times$ 60 min/hr
= 60 ml/hr

c. Concentration/min

4 mg/min

d. Concentration/hr

4 mg/min $\times$ 60 min/hr
= 240 mg/hr

9. *Concentration of solution*

$$400 \text{ mg} : 250 \text{ ml} : : X \text{ mg} : \text{ml}$$
$$250 \text{ X} = 400$$
$$X = 1.6 \text{ mg}$$

concentration of solution
1.6 mg/ml

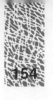

Infusion rates

a. Volume/min

$$60 \text{ ml} : 60 \text{ min} :: X \text{ ml} : \text{min}$$
$$60 X = 60$$
$$X = 1 \text{ ml}$$
$$1 \text{ ml/min}$$

b. Volume/hr

60 ml/hr

c. Concentration/min

$$1.6 \text{ mg/ml} \times 1 \text{ ml/min}$$
$$= 1.6 \text{ mg/min}$$

d. Concentration/hr

$$1.6 \text{ mg/ml} \times 60 \text{ min/hr}$$
$$= 96 \text{ mg/hr}$$

10. *Concentration of solution*

$$4 \text{ mg} = 4000 \text{ mcg}$$
$$4000 \text{ mcg} : 500 \text{ ml} :: X \text{ mcg} : \text{ml}$$
$$500 X = 4000$$
$$X = 8 \text{ mcg}$$

concentration of solution
8 mcg/ml

Infusion rates

a. Volume/min

$$65 \text{ ml} : 60 \text{ min} :: X \text{ ml} : \text{min}$$
$$60 X = 65$$
$$X = 1.083 \text{ ml}$$
$$1.08 \text{ ml/min}$$

b. Volume/hr

65 ml/hr

c. Concentration/min

$$8 \text{ mcg/ml} \times 1.08 \text{ ml/min}$$
$$= 8.64 \text{ mcg/min}$$

d. Concentration/hr

$$8.64 \text{ mcg/min} \times 60 \text{ min/hr}$$
$$= 518.4 \text{ mcg/hr}$$

CALCULATING INFUSION RATES OF A DRUG FOR SPECIFIC BODY WEIGHT PER UNIT TIME

The last method is calculating infusion rates for the amount of drug per unit time for a specific body weight. The weight parameter is an accurate means of dosing for a therapeutic effect. The physician orders the *desired dose per kilogram of body weight* and the *concentration of the solution.* From this information infusion rates can be calculated for administering an individualized dose. Accurate daily weights are essential for the correct dosage.

The previous methods for calculating *concentration of solution* and *infusion rates* for concentration and volume are used with one addition. The *concentration per minute* is obtained by multiplying the *body weight* by the *desired dose per kilogram per minute* and must be done before calculating the other infusion rates.

Currently volumetric pumps do not infuse fractional portions of a milliliter, for example, 1.08 ml/hr. Therefore, if the volume per hour is a fractional amount, it must be rounded off to a whole number, 1.8 ml/hr = 2 ml/hr. When calculating concentration per minute and hour and volume per minute, carry out the problem three decimal places, if necessary, before rounding off. The volume per hour, if fractional, may then be rounded off, making the volume per hour as accurate as possible. There are two exceptions to rounding off fractional infusion rates. If the patient's condition is labile, the difference between 1 or 2 ml could be important. Since physicians order the medication, they must be consulted if any question of drug dosage arises.

A basic fractional equation is given at the end of this section. It can be used as a quick reference only if two of the quantities are known. The basic fractional equation is not as accurate to the nearest hundredth as the other method in this section.

Units/Kilogram Body Weight

Unlike the previous problems, the first step involves determining the desired dose per kilogram per minute, which will be the concentration per minute.

EXAMPLE

Problem: Infuse heparin 5000 units in D_5W 250 ml at 0.15 units/kg/min. Patient weighs 70 kg.

The concentration of solution is 20 units/ml.

How many units/kg would infuse per minute? Per hour?

Find concentration/minute.

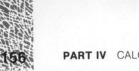

METHOD: **units/min**

Multiply the patient's weight by the desired dose of units/ kg/min.	70 kg × 0.15 units/kg/min = 10.5 units/min

Find concentration/hour.

METHOD: **units/hr**

Multiply the concentration/min by 60 min/hr.	10.5 units/min × 60 min/hr = 630 units/hr

> *Answer:*   The concentration of heparin infused per minute is *10.5 units/min* and per hour is *630 units/hr* for the patient's body weight.

How many milliliters would infuse over one minute? One hour?

Find volume/minute.

METHOD: **ml/min**

Divide the concentration/min by the concentration of the solution.	$\dfrac{10.5 \text{ units/min}}{20 \text{ units/ml}} = 0.5 \text{ ml/min}$

Find volume/hour.

METHOD: **ml/hr**

Multiply the volume/min by 60 min/hr.	0.5 ml/min × 60 min/hr = 30 ml/hr

> *Answer:*   The volume per minute of heparin infused is *0.5 ml/min.* The volume per hour is *30 ml/hr.*

Milligrams/Kilogram Body Weight

EXAMPLE

Problem: Infuse lidocaine 2 g in D$_5$W 500 ml at 0.027 mg/kg/min. Patient weighs 165 lb.

Concentration of solution is lidocaine 4 mg/ml.

How many milligrams/kg would infuse per minute? Per hour?

Convert lb to kg.

Divide lb by 2.2.	$\dfrac{165 \text{ lb}}{2.2 \text{ kg}} = 75 \text{ kg}$

Find concentration/minute.

METHOD: **mg/min**

Multiply the patient's weight by the desired dose of mg/kg/min.	$75 \text{ kg} \times 0.027 \text{ mg/kg/min}$ $= 2.025 \text{ mg/min}$

Find concentration/hour.

METHOD: **mg/hr**

Multiply the concentration/min by 60 min/hr.	$2.025 \text{ mg/min} \times 60 \text{ min/hr} =$ 122 mg/hr

Answer: The concentration of lidocaine infused per minute is *2.025 mg/min* and per hour is *122 mg/hr* for the patient's body weight.

How many milliliters would infuse over one minute? One hour?

Find volume/minute.

METHOD: **ml/min**

Divide the concentration/min by the concentration of the solution.	$\dfrac{2 \text{ mg/min}}{4 \text{ mg/ml}} = 0.5 \text{ ml/min}$

Find volume/hour.

METHOD: **ml/hr**

Multiply the concentration/min by 60 min/hr.	$0.5 \text{ ml/min} \times 60 \text{ min/hr} =$ 30 ml/hr

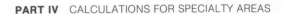

Answer: The volume of lidocaine infused per minute is *0.5 ml/min.* The hourly infusion rate is *30 ml/hr.*

Micrograms/Kilogram Body Weight

EXAMPLE

Problem: Infuse Isuprel 2 mg in 500 ml D₅W at 0.084 mcg/kg/min. Patient weighs 130 lb.

Concentration of solution is 4 mcg/ml.

How many micrograms of Isuprel would be infused per minute? Per hour?

Convert lb to kg.

Divide lb by 2.2.	$\dfrac{130\ lb}{2.2\ kg} = 59.09\ kg$

Find concentration/minute.

METHOD: **mcg/min**

Multiply patient's weight times the desired dose of mcg/kg/min.	59.09 kg × 0.084 mcg/kg/min = 4.964 mcg/min

Find concentration/hour.

METHOD: **mg/hr**

Multiply concentration/min by 60 min/hr.	4.964 mcg/min × 60 min/hr = 297.84 mcg/hr

Answer: The concentration of Isuprel infused per minute and hour is *4.964 mcg/min* and *297.84 mcg/hr* for the patient's body weight.

How many milliliters of Isuprel will infuse per minute? Per hour?

Find volume/minute.

METHOD: **ml/min**

| Divide the concentration/min by the concentration of the solution. | $\dfrac{4.964 \text{ mcg/min}}{4 \text{ mcg/ml}} = 1.241 \text{ ml/min}$ |

Find volume/hour.

METHOD: **ml/hr**

| Multiply volume/min by 60 min/hr. | 1.241 ml/min $\times$ 60 min/hr $= 74.46$ or 74 ml/hr |

> *Answer:* The volume of Isuprel infused per minute is *1.241 ml/min* and the infusion rate per hour is *74 ml/hr*.

Basic Fractional Equation

A basic fractional equation can be used to determine any *one* of the following quantities: concentration of solution, volume per hour, or desired concentration per minute. The equation has one constant, the drop rate of the IV set, 60 gtts/ml. The unknown quantity can be represented by X. (Refer to Chapter 3 for fractional equations.)

$$\frac{\text{concentration of solution (units, mg, mcg/ml)}}{\text{drop rate of set (60 gtts/ml)}} = \frac{\text{desired concentration/min}}{\text{volume/hr (ml/hr) or gtts/min}}$$

1. Use the formula to find the volume/hr or gtts/min.

EXAMPLE

Infuse heparin 5000 units in D_5W in 250 ml at 0.15 units/kg/min. Patient weighs 70 kg. The concentration of solution is 20 units/ml.

desired concentration/minute: 0.15 units/kg/min $\times$ 70 kg = 10.5 units/min

$$\frac{20 \text{ units/ml}}{60 \text{ gtts/ml}} = \frac{10.5 \text{ units/min}}{\text{X (ml/hr or gtts/min)}}$$

20 X = 630

X = 31 ml/hr or 31 gtts/min

(On page 156, the answer is 30 ml/hr.)

2. Use the formula to find the desired concentration/minute.

EXAMPLE

Infuse lidocaine 2 g in D_5W 500 ml with a rate of 30 ml/hr. The concentration of solution is 4 mg/ml.

$$\frac{4 \text{ mg/ml}}{60 \text{ gtts/ml}} = \frac{X}{30 \text{ ml/hr}}$$

$$60 \text{ X} = 120$$
$$\text{X} = 2 \text{ mg/min (On page 157, the answer}$$
$$\text{is 2 mg/min.)}$$

3. Use the formula to find the concentration of solution.

EXAMPLE

Infuse Isuprel 2 mg in 500 ml D_5W at 0.084 mcg/kg/min with rate of 74 ml/hr. Patient weighs 59 kg.

$$\text{desired concentration/minute} = 0.084 \text{ mcg/kg/min} \times 59 \text{ kg} =$$
$$4.95 \text{ mcg/min}$$

$$\frac{X}{60 \text{ gtts/ml}} = \frac{4.95 \text{ mcg/min}}{74 \text{ ml/hr}}$$

$$74 \text{ X} = 297$$
$$\text{X} = 4 \text{ mcg/ml (On page 143, the answer}$$
$$\text{is 4 mcg/ml.)}$$

Practice Problems

Determine the infusion rates for specific body weight by calculating the following:

- Concentration of solution
- Weight in kilograms
- Infusion rates
  a. concentration/minute
  b. concentration/hour (not always measured)
  c. volume/minute
  d. volume/hour

You may use the basic fractional formula and compare answers.

1. Infuse dobutamine 500 mg in 250 ml D$_5$W at 5 mcg/kg/min. Patient weighs 182 lb.

_____

2. Infuse amrinone 250 mg in 250 ml NS at 5 mcg/kg/min. Patient weighs 165 lb.

_____

3. Infuse dopamine 400 mg in 250 ml D$_5$W at 10 mcg/kg/min. Patient weighs 140 lb.

_____

4. Infuse nitroprusside 100 mg in 500 ml D$_5$W at 3 mcg/kg/min. Patient weighs 55 kg.

_____

5. Infuse dobutamine 1000 mg in 500 ml D$_5$W at 15 mcg/kg/min. Patient weighs 110 lb.

ANSWERS

1. Infuse dobutamine 500 mg in 250 ml D$_5$W at 5 mcg/kg/min. Patient weighs 182 lb.

Concentration of solution   _lb to kg_

$$500 \text{ mg} = 500,000 \text{ mcg}$$
$$500,000 : 250 \text{ ml} :: X \text{ mcg} : \text{ml}$$
$$250 \text{ X} = 500,000$$
$$X = 2000 \text{ mcg}$$

$$\frac{182}{2.2} = 82.7 \text{ kg}$$

concentration of solution is 2000 mcg/ml

Infusion rates

a. Concentration/min

Pt weight $\times$ Desired dose/kg/min
82.7 kg $\times$ 5 mcg/kg/min
= 413.5 mcg/min

b. Concentration/hr

413.5 mcg/min $\times$
60 min/hr =
24,810 mcg/hr

c. Volume/min

$$\frac{413.5 \text{ mcg/min}}{2000 \text{ mcg/ml}} = 0.206 \text{ ml/min}$$

d. Volume/hr

0.206 ml/min × 60 min/hr
= 12.36 or 12 ml/hr

2. Infuse amrinone 250 mg in 250 ml NS at 5 mcg/kg/min. Patient weighs 165 lb.

Concentration of solution   *lb to kg*

250 mg = 250,000 mcg $\dfrac{165}{2.2} = 75$ kg
250,000 mcg : 250 ml : : X mcg : ml
250 X = 250,000
X = 1000 mcg

concentration of solution is 1000 mcg/ml

Infusion rates

a. Concentration/min

Pt weight × Desired dose/kg/min
75 kg × 5 mcg/kg/min = 375 mcg/min

b. Concentration/hr

375 mcg/min ×
60 min/hr =
22,500 mcg/hr

c. Volume/min

$$\dfrac{375 \text{ mcg/min}}{1000 \text{ mcg/ml}} = 0.375 \text{ ml/min}$$

d. Volume/hr

0.375 ml/min × 60 min/hr
= 22.5 ml/hr or
23 ml/hr

3. Infuse dopamine 400 mg in 250 ml D$_5$W at 10 mcg/kg/min. Patient weighs 140 lb.

Concentration of solution   *lb to kg*

400 mg = 400,000 mcg $\dfrac{140}{2.2} = 63.6$ kg
400,000 mg : 250 ml = X mg : ml
250 X = 400,000
X = 1600 mcg

concentration of solution is 1600 mcg/ml

Infusion rates

a. Concentration/min

Pt weight × Desired dose/kg/min
63.6 kg × 10 mcg/kg/min
= 636 mcg/min

b. Concentration/hr

636 mcg/min ×
60 min/hr =
38,160 mcg/hr

c. Volume/min

$$\frac{636 \text{ mcg/min}}{1600 \text{ mcg/ml}} = 0.39 \text{ ml/min}$$

d. Volume/hr

0.39 ml/min × 60 min/hr
= 23.4 ml/hr
or 23 ml/hr

4. Infuse nitroprusside 100 mg in 500 ml D_5W at 3 mcg/min. Patient weighs 55 kg.

Concentration of solution *Patient weighs*

100 mg = 100,000 mcg 55 kg
100,000 mcg : 500 ml : : X mg : ml
500 X = 100,000
X = 200 mcg

concentration of solution is 200 mcg/ml

Infusion rates

a. Concentration/min

3 mcg/kg/min × 55 kg =
165 mcg/min

b. Concentration/hr

165 mcg/min × 60 min/hr =
9900 mcg/hr

c. Volume/min

$$\frac{165 \text{ mcg/min}}{200 \text{ mcg/ml}} = 0.825 \text{ ml/min}$$

d. Volume/hr

0.825 ml/min $\times$ 60 min/hr = 49.5 ml/hr or 50 ml/hr

5. Infuse dobutamine 1000 mg in 500 ml D$_5$W at 15 mcg/kg/min. Patient weighs 110 lb.

Concentration of solution   *lb to kg*

$$1000 \text{ mg} = 1{,}000{,}000 \text{ mcg}$$
$$1{,}000{,}000 \text{ mg} : 500 \text{ ml} = X : \text{ml}$$
$$500 \text{ X} = 1{,}000{,}000$$
$$X = 2000 \text{ mcg}$$

$$\frac{110}{2.2} = 50 \text{ kg}$$

concentration of solution is 2000 mcg/ml

Infusion rates

a. Concentration/min

Pt weight $\times$ Desired dose/kg/min
50 kg $\times$ 15 mcg/kg/min
= 750 mcg/min

b. Concentration/hr

750 mcg/min $\times$
60 min/hr =
45,000 mcg/hr

c. Volume/min

$$\frac{750 \text{ mcg/min}}{2000 \text{ mcg/ml}} = 0.375 \text{ ml/min}$$

d. Volume/hr

0.375 ml/min $\times$ 60 min/hr
= 22.5 ml/hr
or 23 ml/hr

TITRATION OF INFUSION RATE

Drugs administered by titration are based on *concentration of solution, infusion rates, specific concentration per kilogram of body weight,* and *titration factor.* The titration factor is the concentration of drug per drop, units/gtt, mg/gtt, or mcg/gtt. The titration factor can be added to or subtracted from the baseline infusion rate to determine the exact concentration of an infusion. Since the titration method of drug administration is primarily used when a patient's condition is labile, calculating the titration factor will give the nurse the means for determining the exact amount of drug infusing.

Charts for drug infusion, developed by drug manufacturers, can be used for adjusting infusion rates for drug titrations. Often the amount of drug being infused falls between calibrations on the charts. When that occurs, the titration factor can be used to determine the exact concentration of drug being administered. The titration factor can also be used to verify the correct selection from the chart.

EXAMPLE

Isuprel 2 mg in 250 ml D_5W.

Titrate 1 mcg–3 mcg/min to maintain HR (heart rate) > 50, < 130 and B/P > 90 systolic.

A. Concentration of solution

Convert mg to mcg. Set up ratio/proportion.	2 mg = 2000 mcg 2000 mcg : 250 ml : : X mcg : ml 250 X = 2000 X = 8 mcg 8 mcg/ml

B. Infusion rate by volume/unit time

Desired infusion rate by concentration is stated in the problem. Note that the upper dosage and lower dosage must be determined.

Remember: Hourly rate and the number of gtts per minute are the same with a microdrip administration set.

Volume rate/minute: ml/min

	Lower	Upper
Divide concentration/min by concentration of solution.	$\dfrac{1 \text{ mcg/min}}{8 \text{ mcg/ml}} =$	$\dfrac{3 \text{ mcg/min}}{8 \text{ mcg/ml}} =$
	0.125 ml/min	0.375 ml/min

Volume rate/hour: ml/hr (equivalent to gtts/min)

Lower

Volume rate/min Multiply × 60 min.	0.125 ml/min × 60 = 7.5 ml/hr (7.5 gtts/min)

Upper

0.375 ml/hr × 60 min/hr =
22.5 ml/hr (22.5 gtts/min)

C. The titration factor

Find: Rate in gtts/min. Divide: Concentration/min by gtts/min.

7.5 gtts/min

$$\frac{1 \text{ mcg/min}}{7.5 \text{ gtts/min}} =$$

0.133 mcg/gtt

The *titration factor* is 0.133 mcg/gtt in a solution of Isuprel labeled 2 mg in 250 ml D₅W. To repeat, changing drops/minute results in a corresponding change in ml/hr. If the baseline infusion rates are **1 mcg/min** for concentration and **7.5 ml/hr** for volume, increasing the infusion rate by **1 gtt/min** changes the concentration/minute by **0.133 mcg** and increases the hourly volume by **1 ml** to give a rate of **8.5 ml/hr.**

D. Increasing/decreasing rates

To increase the infusion rate by 5 gtts/min, from a baseline rate of 1 mcg/min, set up a ratio/proportion or multiply the titration factor (mcg/gtt) by 5 to obtain the increment of increase.

EXAMPLE

Set up a ratio/proportion with rate in gtts/min as the known variables.

7.5 gtts : 1 mcg : : 5 gtts : X mcg
      7.5 X = 5
         X = 0.666 mcg
           5 gtts/0.66 mcg

or

Multiply titration factor, mcg/gtt × 5.

0.133 mcg/gtt × 5 gtts
  = 0.665 mcg

By adding 5 gtts/min, the volume infusion rate has increased 5 ml/hr, from 7.5 ml/hr to 12.5 ml/hr. The concentration of drug delivered is increased by 0.665 mcg/min to 1.665 mcg/min.

Ex.   1.000 mcg/min   Baseline rate
    + 0.665 mcg/min   Increment of rate increased
     1.665 mcg/min   Adjusted infusion rate

Suppose the infusion rate was 3 mcg/min and a decrease was needed. To decrease the infusion rate by 10 gtts, set up another ratio/proportion or multiply the titration factor (mcg/gtt) by 10.

EXAMPLE

Set up a ratio/proportion with rate in gtts/mcg as the known variables.	7.5 gtts : 1 mcg = 10 gtts : X mcg 7.5 X = 10 X = 1.33 mcg 1.33 mcg/10 gtts

or

Multiply titration factor, mcg/gtt × 10.	0.133 mcg/gtt × 10 gtts = 1.33 mcg

By subtracting 10 gtts/min, the infusion rate has decreased 10 ml/hr from 22.5 ml/hr to 12.5 ml/hr. The amount of drug delivered is decreased by 1.33 mcg/min to 1.67 mcg/min.

Ex.

	3.00 mcg/min	Baseline infusion rate
−	1.33 mcg/min	Increment of rate decreased
	1.67 mcg/min	Adjusted infusion rate

Practice Problems with Answers

1. Nitroprusside 50 mg in 250 ml D_5W. Titrate 0.5–1.5 mcg/kg/min to maintain mean B/P at 100 mm Hg. Patient weighs 70 kg.

   Find the following:

   a. Concentration of solution

   _____

   b. Concentration/minute

   _____

   c. Volume/minute and hour

   _____

   d. Titration factor

   _____

   e. Increase the infusion rate of 11 gtts/min by 5 gtts. What is the concentration/minute? What is the volume/hour?

   _____

   f. Increase the infusion rate from 16 gtts/ml by 13 gtts. What is the concentration/minute? What is the volume/hour?

   _____

ANSWER

a. Concentration of solution

$$50 \text{ mg} = 50,000 \text{ mcg}$$
$$50,000 \text{ mcg} : 250 \text{ ml} : : X \text{ mcg} : 1 \text{ ml}$$
$$250 X = 50,000$$
$$X = 200 \text{ mcg}$$

concentration of solution is 200 mcg/ml

b. Concentration/minute

Lower: 0.5 mcg/kg/min $\times$ 70 kg = 35 mcg/min

Upper: 1.5 mcg/kg/min $\times$ 70 kg = 105 mcg/min

c. Volume/minute and hour

Lower: $\dfrac{35 \text{ mcg/min}}{200 \text{ mcg/ml}}$ = 0.175 ml/min $\times$ 60 min/hr = 10.5 or 11 ml/hr

Upper: $\dfrac{105 \text{ mcg/min}}{200 \text{ mcg/ml}}$ = 0.525 ml/min $\times$ 60 min/hr = 31.5 or 32 ml/hr

d. Titration factor

11 ml/hr = 11 gtts/min $\dfrac{35 \text{ mcg/min}}{11 \text{ gtts/min}}$ = 3.18 or 3 mcg/gtt

e. Increase the infusion rate of 11 gtts/min by 5 gtts. What is the concentration/minute? What is the volume/hour?

$$5 \text{ gtts} \times 3 \text{ mcg/gtt} = 15 \text{ mcg}$$
$$15 \text{ mcg} + 35 \text{ mcg/min} = 50 \text{ mcg/min}$$
$$5 \text{ gtts} + 11 \text{ gtts/min} = 16 \text{ gtts/min or } 16 \text{ ml/hr}$$

f. Increase the infusion rate from 16 gtts/ml by 13 gtts. What is the concentration/minute? What is the volume/hour?

13 gtts $\times$ 3 mcg/gtt = 39 mcg   39 mcg + 50 mcg = 89 mcg/min

13 gtts + 16 gtts = 29 gtts/ml or 29 ml/hr

2. Dopamine 400 mg in 250 ml D_5W. Titrate beginning at 4 mcg/kg/min to maintain a mean B/P of 100 to 120 systolic. Patient weighs 75 kg. Find the following:

a. Concentration of solution

_____

b. Concentration/minute

_____

c. Volume/minute and hour

_____

d. Titration factor

_____

e. Increase the infusion rate from 113 gtts/min by 7 gtts. What is the concentration/minute? What is the volume/hour?

_____

f. Decrease the infusion rate from 120 ml/hr (120 gtts/min) by 5 gtts. What is the concentration/minute? What is the volume/hour?

_____

ANSWER

a. Concentration of solution

$$400 \text{ mg} = 40{,}000 \text{ mcg}$$
$$40{,}000 \text{ mcg} : 250 \text{ ml} :: X \text{ mcg} : 1 \text{ ml}$$
$$250 \text{ X} = 40{,}000 \text{ mcg}$$
$$X = 160 \text{ mcg}$$

concentration of solution is 160 mcg/ml

b. Concentration/minute

$$4 \text{ mcg/kg/min} \times 75 \text{ kg} = 300 \text{ mcg/min}$$

c. Volume/minute and hour

$$\frac{300 \text{ mcg/min}}{160 \text{ mcg/ml}} = 1.875 \text{ ml/min} \times 60 \text{ min/hr} = 112.5$$
$$\text{or } 113 \text{ ml/hr}$$

d. Titration factor

$$113 \text{ ml/hr} = 113 \text{ gtts/min}$$

$$\frac{300 \text{ mcg/min}}{113 \text{ gtts/min}} = 2.65 \text{ or } 3 \text{ mcg/gtt}$$

e. Increase the infusion rate from 113 gtts/min by 7 gtts. What is the concentration/minute? What is the volume/hour?

$$7 \text{ gtts} \times 3 \text{ mcg/gtts} = 21 \text{ mcg}$$

$$21 \text{ mcg} + 300 \text{ mcg/min} = 321 \text{ mcg/min}$$

$$7 \text{ gtts} + 113 \text{ gtts/min} = 120 \text{ gtts/min or } 120 \text{ ml/hr}$$

f. Decrease the infusion rate from 120 ml/hr (120 gtts/min) by 5 gtts. What is the concentration/minute? What is the volume/hour?

$$5 \text{ gtts} \times 3 \text{ mcg/gtts} = 15 \text{ mcg}$$

$$321 \text{ mcg/min} - 15 \text{ mcg} = 306 \text{ mcg/min}$$

$$120 \text{ gtts/min} - 5 \text{ gtts} = 115 \text{ gtts/min or } 115 \text{ ml/hr}$$

TOTAL AMOUNT OF DRUG INFUSED OVER TIME

Determining the total amount of drug infused over time is useful when changes in drug therapy occur. If adverse effects, toxic levels, therapeutic failure, or discontinuance of a drug occurs, knowing the amount that was administered can be important for charting and future therapies.

For this calculation, the concentration of the drug in solution must be known, as must the time that drug therapy began to the nearest minute. Again, with 60 gtt sets, the hourly rate is the same as the drip rate per minute.

EXAMPLE

Heparin 10,000 units in 250 ml D_5W at 30 ml/hr has been infusing for 3 hours. The drug was discontinued.

How much heparin did the patient receive?

Concentration of solution

Set up a ratio/proportion. Solve for X.	10,000 units : 250 ml : : X units : ml $250\ X = 10,000$ $X = 40$ units 40 units/ml

Concentration/hour

Multiply concentration of solution by volume/hr.	40 units/ml $\times$ 30 ml/hr $= 1200$ units/hr

Total amount of drug infused

Multiply concentration/hr by length of administration.	1200 units/hr $\times$ 3 hr $= 3600$ units/3 hr

Answer: The total amount of heparin that infused over 3 hours was 3600 units.

Practice Problems with Answers

Solve for the amount of drug infused over time.

1. In one hour, a patient received two boluses of lidocaine 100 mg and an IV infusion of 4 mg/ml at 40 ml/hr for 30 min. How many mg have infused?

NOTE: Do not exceed 300 mg/hr of lidocaine.

ANSWER

Lidocaine bolus: 100 mg
<u>100</u> mg
200 mg

Lidocaine IV infusion:

A. Concentration of solution: Given 4 mg/ml in problem.

B. Concentration/hr

$$4 \text{ mg/ml} \times 40 \text{ ml/hr} = 160 \text{ mg/hr}$$

C. Concentration over ½ hr

$$160 \text{ mg/hr} \times \frac{30 \text{ min}}{60 \text{ min/hr}} = 80 \text{ mg over 30 min}$$

D. Amount of IV drug infused

Lidocaine per 2 boluses: 200 mg
Lidocaine per IV infusion: <u>80</u> mg
280 mg total amount infused
over 1 hr

NOTE: The infusion rate is close to exceeding the maximum therapeutic range, which is 200–300 mg/hr.

2. Heparin 20,000 units in 500 ml D_5W at 50 ml/hr has been infusing for 5 ½ hours. The drug has been discontinued. How much heparin has been given?

ANSWER

Concentration of solution

20,000 units : 500 ml : : X units : 1 ml
500 X = 20,000
X = 40 units

concentration of solution is 40 units/ml
Concentration/hr

$$40 \text{ units/ml} \times 50 \text{ ml/hr} = 2000 \text{ units/hr}$$

Amount of IV drug infused over 5 ½ hours

$$2000 \text{ units} \times \frac{30 \text{ min}}{60 \text{ min/hr}} = 1000 \text{ units over } \tfrac{1}{2} \text{ hr}$$

$$2000 \text{ units} \times 5 \text{ hr} \qquad = 10,000 \text{ units/5 hr}$$

10,000 units
<u>1,000 units</u>
11,000 units over 5 ½ hr

FACTORS INFLUENCING INTRAVENOUS ADMINISTRATION
CALCULATING ACCURACY OF DILUTION PARAMETERS

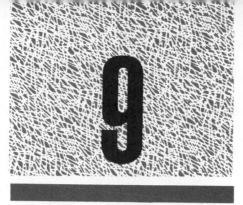

C H A P T E R

Pediatric Critical Care

Objectives

- Recognize factors that contribute to errors in drug and fluid administration.
- Identify the steps in calculating dilution parameters.
- Determine the accuracy of the dilution parameters in a drug order.

In delivering emergency drugs with complex dilution calculations, it is important for the nurse to evaluate the accuracy of the physician's order and ensure that the child does not receive excessive fluids. Many institutions are attempting to standardize the concentration of the solution for various pediatric intravenous dosages to decrease miscalculations.

As noted in Chapter 8, the concepts of concentration of the solution, infusion rates for concentration and volume, and concentration of a drug for specific body weight per unit time are also used to prepare the pediatric dose.

FACTORS INFLUENCING INTRAVENOUS ADMINISTRATION

Excessive fluid can be given when the fluid volume of the emergency drug is not considered in the 24-hour fluid intake. Long intravenous tubing can be another source of fluid excess and can cause errors in drug delivery. When the priming or filling volume of the intravenous tubing is not considered, the child may receive extra fluid, especially if medication is added to the primary IV set via a secondary IV set. Intravenous medication may not reach the child if the IV infusion rate is low, such as 1 ml/hr, and the IV tubing has not been primed or filled with the medication prior to infusion. Most pediatric areas are developing protocol for safe and consistent IV drug delivery.

CALCULATING ACCURACY OF DILUTION PARAMETERS

The nurse may find it necessary to calculate the dilution parameters of a drug order that specifies the concentration/kg/minute and the volume/hour infusion rate. The physician should determine all drug dose parameters, which include concentration/kg/minute, volume/hour, and dilution parameters. The nurse should check the accuracy of the dilution parameters to ensure that the correct drug dosage is given. The methods used below are also used to prepare the pediatric dose. In many pediatric critical care areas, intravenous fluids for drug administration are limited to prevent fluid overload. If the physician changes the drug dosage, rather than increase the volume (ml), the concentration of the solution may be changed.

EXAMPLES

Problem 1:   A 6-day-old infant, weight 3.5 kg, is in septic shock.

Order: dopamine 5 mcg/kg/min at 1 ml/hr and dilute as follows, 100 mg in 100 ml D_5 ½ NS.

Dosage: 2–5 mcg/kg/min.

Drug available: dopamine 40 mg/ml.

The following steps are needed to determine if dilution orders will give the correct concentration of solution to deliver 5 mcg/kg/min at 1 ml/hr.

Step 1:   Determine infusion rates for concentration/unit time.

1. Find the concentration/minute.

Infant weight × concentration/kg/min =
3.5 kg   ×   5 mcg/kg/min   = 17.5 mcg/min

2. Calculate the concentration/hour.

17.5 mcg/min × 60 min/hr = 1050 mcg/hr

Step 2:   Determine concentration of solution.

Divide the concentration/hr by volume/hr.

$$\frac{1050 \text{ mcg/hr}}{1 \text{ ml/hr}} = 1050 \text{ mcg/ml or } 1 \text{ mg/ml}$$

Step 3:   Determine accuracy of dilution order.

Find how much dopamine must be added to 100 ml.

Set up a ratio and proportion.

1 mg : 1 ml = X : 100 ml
X = 100 mg

Dilution order is correct/accurate.

Preparation of Drug Dosage:

$$\frac{D}{H} \times V = \frac{100}{40} \times 1 = 2.5 \text{ ml or}$$

mg	ml		mg	ml
H	: V	::	D	: V
40	: 1	::	100	: X

40 X = 100
X = 2.5 ml

Answer: Add 2.5 ml of dopamine 40 mg/ml to 100 ml D_5 ½ NS.

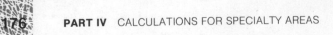

Problem 2:   A 3-week-old infant, weight 1.6 kg, in septic shock.

Order: dobutamine 2.5 mcg/kg/min by a syringe pump with a 35 ml syringe at 1 ml/hr.

Dilution: dobutamine 8.4 mg with D_5 ¼ NS to equal 35 ml.

Dosage: 2.5 mcg/kg/min to 40 mcg/kg/min.

Drug available: dobutamine 250 mg/20 ml.

Determine accuracy of dilution order to deliver 2.5 mcg/kg/min at 1 ml/hr.

Step 1:   Infusion rates for concentration/unit time.

1. Concentration/minute.

Infant weight × concentration/kg/min =
1.6 kg   ×   2.5 mcg/kg/min   =   4 mcg/min

2. Concentration/hour.

4 mcg/min × 60 min/hr = 240 mcg/hr

Step 2:   Concentration of solution.

Divide the concentration/hr by volume/hr.

$$\frac{240 \text{ mcg/hr}}{1 \text{ ml/hr}} = 240 \text{ mcg/ml}$$

Step 3:   Accuracy of dilution order.

Find how much dobutamine must be added to make 35 ml.

```
mcg     ml      mcg      ml
240  :  1  ::   X    :   35
            X = 8400 mcg or 8.4 mg
```

Dilution order is correct/accurate.

Preparation of Drug Dosage:

$$\frac{D}{H} = \frac{8.4 \text{ mg}}{250 \text{ mg}} \times 20 \text{ ml} = 0.672 \text{ ml}$$

or

```
mg  :  ml  ::  mg  :  ml
250  :  20  ::  8.4  :  X
        250 X = 168
           X = 0.67 ml
```

Answer: Add 0.67 ml of dobutamine 250 mg/20 ml to 34.33 ml D_5 ¼ NS.

Problem 3: For the same infant the physician increases dobutamine. Again fluids must be limited and another concentration must be prepared.

Order: 15 mcg/kg/min, deliver in syringe pump. Dilute 40.5 mg in 35 ml D_5 ¼ NS and administer 1 ml/hr.

Determine accuracy of dilution order to deliver 15 mcg/kg/min at 1 ml/hr.

Step 1: Infusion rates for concentration/unit time.

1. Concentration/minute.

Infant's weight × concentration/kg/min =
$$1.6 \text{ kg} \quad \times \quad 15 \text{ mcg/kg/min} \quad = \quad 24 \text{ mcg/min}$$

2. Concentration/hour.

$$24 \text{ mcg/min} \times 60 \text{ min/hr} = 1440 \text{ mcg/hr}$$

Step 2: Concentration of solution.

Divide the concentration/hr by volume/hr.

$$\frac{1440 \text{ mcg/hr}}{1 \text{ ml/hr}} = 1440 \text{ mcg/ml}$$

Step 3: Accuracy of dilution order.

$$
\begin{array}{ccccccc}
\text{mcg} & : & \text{ml} & :: & \text{mcg} & : & \text{ml} \\
1440 & : & 1 & :: & X & : & 35 \\
\end{array}
$$
$$X = 50,400 \text{ mcg}$$

or

$$50.4 \text{ mg}$$

or

$$50 \text{ mg}$$

The dilution order is *incorrect*; 50 mg of dobutamine is needed to deliver 15 mcg/kg/min.

SUMMARY PRACTICE PROBLEMS

Determine if dilution orders will yield the correct concentration of solution.

1. A 2-year-old is being treated for acute status asthmaticus.
Child weighs 10.5 kg.

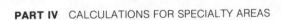

Order: Aminophyllin 110 mg in 500 ml at 40 ml/hr.

Pediatric dose: 0.85 mg/kg/hr.

Drug available: Aminophyllin 250 mg/10 ml.

2. A 9-year-old child with supraventricular tachycardia.

Child weighs 30 kg.

Order: lidocaine 20 mcg/kg/min.

  Dilute: 300 mg in 250 ml of D₅W at 30 ml/hr.

Pediatric dose: 20–40 mcg/kg/min.

Drug available: lidocaine 1 g/25 ml.

3. A 1-year-old child with septic shock.

Child weighs 9 kg.

Order: dopamine 5 mcg/kg/min.

  Dilute: 100 mg in 200 ml of D₅ ¼ NS at 6.75 ml/hr.

Pediatric dose: 2–5 mcg/kg/min.

Drug available: dopamine 400 mg/5 ml.

4. A 3-year-old child in shock.

Child weighs 16 kg.

Order: sodium nitroprusside 2 mcg/kg/min.

Dilute 25.25 mg in 250 D$_5$W at 19 ml/hr.

Pediatric dose: 200–500 mcg/kg/hr.

Drug available: sodium nitroprusside 50 mg/5 ml.

ANSWERS

1. Step 1:   Infusion rates—concentration.

      a. Concentration/hour

$$10.5 \text{ kg} \times 0.85 \text{ mg/kg/hr} = 8.9 \text{ mg/hr}$$

Step 2:   Concentration of solution.

$$\frac{8.9 \text{ mg/hr}}{40 \text{ ml/hr}} = 0.22 \text{ mg/ml}$$

Step 3:   Accuracy of dilution order.

$$
\begin{array}{ccccccc}
\text{mg} & : & \text{ml} & :: & \text{mg} & : & \text{ml} \\
0.22 & : & 1 & :: & X & : & 500 \\
& & & X = 110 \text{ mg} & & &
\end{array}
$$

Dilution order is correct/accurate.

Preparation of Drug Dosage:

$$\frac{D}{H} = \frac{110}{250} \times 10 = \frac{1100}{250} = 4.4 \text{ ml}$$

or

$$
\begin{array}{ccccccc}
\text{mg} & : & \text{ml} & :: & \text{mg} & : & \text{ml} \\
250 & : & 10 & :: & 110 & : & X \\
& & 250\,X = 1100 & & & & \\
& & X = 4.4 \text{ ml} & & & &
\end{array}
$$

Answer: 4.4 ml of Aminophyllin to be added to 500 ml.

2. Step 1: Infusion rates for concentration/unit time.

        a. Concentration/minute

$$30 \text{ kg} \times 20 \text{ mcg/kg/min} = 600 \text{ mcg/min}$$

        b. Concentration/hour

$$600 \text{ mcg/min} \times 60 \text{ min/hr} = 36,000 \text{ mcg/hr}$$

Step 2: Concentration of solution.

$$\frac{36,000 \text{ mcg/hr}}{30 \text{ ml/hr}} = 1200 \text{ mcg/ml } or \text{ } 1.2 \text{ mg/ml}$$

Step 3: Accuracy of dilution order.

$$
\begin{array}{ccccccc}
\text{mg} & : & \text{ml} & :: & \text{mg} & : & \text{ml} \\
1.2 & : & 1 & :: & \text{X} & : & 250
\end{array}
$$
$$\text{X} = 300 \text{ mg}$$

Dilution order is correct/accurate.

Preparation of Drug Dosage:

$$\frac{\text{D}}{\text{H}} = \frac{300}{1000} \times 25 = \frac{7500}{1000} = 7.5 \text{ ml } \text{ or }
\begin{array}{ccccccc}
\text{mg} & : & \text{ml} & :: & \text{mg} & : & \text{ml} \\
1000 & : & 25 & :: & 300 & : & \text{X}
\end{array}$$
$$1000 \text{ X} = 7500$$
$$\text{X} = 7.5 \text{ ml}$$

Answer: 7.5 ml of lidocaine added to 250 ml.

3. Step 1: Infusion rate for concentration.

        a. Concentration/minute

$$9 \text{ kg} \times 5 \text{ mcg/kg/min} = 45 \text{ mcg/min}$$

        b. Concentration/hour

$$45 \text{ mcg/min} \times 60 \text{ min/hr} = 2700 \text{ mcg/hr}$$

Step 2: Concentration of solution.

$$\frac{2700 \text{ mcg/hr}}{6.75 \text{ ml/hr}} = 400 \text{ mcg/ml}$$

Step 3: Accuracy of dilution order.

$$
\begin{array}{ccccccc}
400 \text{ mcg} & : & 1 \text{ ml} & :: & \text{X} \text{ mcg} & : & 200 \text{ ml}
\end{array}
$$
$$\text{X} = 80,000 \text{ mcg or } 80 \text{ mg in } 200 \text{ ml}$$

Dilution order is incorrect.

Answer: Dopamine 80 mg in 200 ml.

4. Step 1:   Infusion rates—concentration.

> **a.** Concentration/minute
>
> $$16 \text{ kg} \times 2 \text{ mcg/kg/min} = 32 \text{ mcg/min}$$
>
> **b.** Concentration/hour
>
> $$32 \text{ mcg/min} \times 60 \text{ min/hr} = 1920 \text{ mcg/hr}$$

Step 2:   Concentration of solution.

$$\frac{1920 \text{ mcg/hr}}{19 \text{ ml/hr}} = 101 \text{ mcg/ml}$$

Step 3:   Accuracy of order.

> 101 mcg : 1 ml : : X mcg : 250 ml
>
> X = 25,250 mcg or 25.25 mg

Dilution order is correct/accurate.

Preparation of Drug Dosage:

$$\frac{D}{H} \times V = \frac{25.25}{50} \times 5 = 2.52 \text{ ml} \quad or$$

mg   :   ml   : :   mg   :   ml
50 mg : 5 ml : : 25.25 mg : X ml
50 X = 126.25
X = 2.52 ml

Answer: 2.52 ml of sodium nitroprusside added to 250 ml.

FACTORS INFLUENCING IV FLUID AND DRUG MANAGEMENT

TITRATION OF MEDICATIONS WITH MAINTENANCE IV FLUIDS

Administration by Concentration

Administration by Volume

INTRAVENOUS LOADING DOSE

INTRAVENOUS FLUID BOLUS

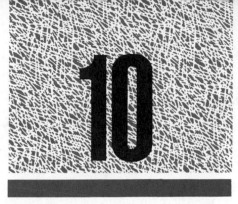

Labor and Delivery

Objectives

- State the complication related to IV fluid administration in the high-risk mother.
- Recognize the different types of fluid administration used in high-risk labors.
- Determine the infusion rates of a drug in solution when the drug is prescribed by concentration or volume.

Drug calculations for labor and delivery are the same as those used in critical care. Determining the concentration of the solution, infusion rates, and titration factors are the primary calculation skills used. Accurate calculations are essential along with the monitoring of intravenous fluid intake for medications and anesthesic procedures. Impaired renal filtration in preeclampsia and the antidiuretic effect of the tocolytic drugs make the monitoring of fluid intake vital. Accurate measurement of intravenous fluid intake along with pulmonary assessment can decrease the risk of fluid overload and the sequelae of acute pulmonary edema in the high-risk mother.

Physicians' orders and hospital protocols give specific guidelines for administering IV drugs. The nurse is responsible for managing the IV drug therapy, monitoring the patient's fluid balance, and assessing response to drug therapy.

FACTORS INFLUENCING IV FLUID AND DRUG MANAGEMENT

The most important concept in labor and delivery is that the drugs given to the mother also affect the unborn baby. Therefore, the response of the patient and the unborn baby must be closely monitored. Vital signs, urine output, reflexes, and contraction patterns are the main indicators of the mother's status. For the fetus, fetal heart rate is the primary guide.

TITRATION OF MEDICATIONS WITH MAINTENANCE IV FLUIDS

Women in labor receive IV fluids to prevent dehydration when oral intake is contraindicated. IV drugs are given to stimulate labor, treat preeclampsia, or inhibit preterm labor. Normally the IV fluids that the patient receives are given at 100 to 125 ml/hr. A bolus of IV fluids, 200 to 500 ml, may be given to initially hydrate the mother, especially in preterm labor, or prior to conductive anesthesia. Any IV medications that are given by titration are a part of the hourly IV rate. The patient will have a primary IV line and a secondary IV line for medications. All IV medications should be delivered by a volumetric pump, which ensures that the specified volume and correct dosage are delivered.

Titration of drugs is frequently done for high-risk mothers with preeclampsia and mothers experiencing preterm labor. The most common use of titration is in the induction or stimulation of labor. In the following example, an oxytocic drug is given and the primary IV rate is adjusted with the secondary IV drug line to achieve a therapeutic effect and maintain adequate maternal hydration. Note that the drug is ordered to be given by concentration and that the infusion rates for volume/minute and hour must be determined.

Administration by Concentration

EXAMPLE

1. Give IV fluids at 100 ml/hr with D_5 ½ NS.
2. Mix 10 units of oxytocin in 1000 NS. Start at 5 mU/minute, increase by 1 or 2 mU/minute, q 10 min, until uterine contractions are 2 to 3 minutes apart, not to exceed 40 mU/minute.

NOTE: 1 Unit (U) = 1000 milliunits (mU)

Available: Secondary Set:
                  Oxytocin 10 units/ml
                  1000 ml NS
                  Microdrip IV set 60 gtts/ml
                  Volumetric pump
           Primary Set:
                  1000 ml D_5 ½ NS
                  IV set drop factor 10 gtts/ml

For the *secondary* set IV, the following calculations must be made:

1. Concentration of solution.
2. Infusion rates: volume/minute and hour.
3. Titration factor in concentration/minute (mU/min).

For the *primary* IV, the following calculations must be made:

1. Drop rate/minute.
2. Balance primary IV flow with secondary IV rate to achieve 100 ml/hr.

Secondary IV (Review Chapter 6 for formulas)

1. Concentration of solution:

$$10 \text{ units} \; : \; 1000 \text{ ml} \; :: \; X \; : \; 1 \text{ ml}$$
$$1000 \, X = 10$$
$$X = 0.01 \text{ units or 10 milliunits}$$

The concentration of solution is 10 mU/ml.

2. Infusion rates for volume:

$$\frac{\text{concentration/minute}}{\text{concentration of sol.}} = \text{volume/minute} \times 60 \text{ minutes} = \text{volume/hour}$$

Volume/minute   *Volume/hour*

$$\frac{1 \text{ mU/minute}}{10 \text{ mU/ml}} = 0.1 \text{ ml/minute} \times 60 \text{ minutes} = 6 \text{ ml/hr}$$

$$\frac{2 \text{ mU/minute}}{10 \text{ mU/ml}} = 0.2 \text{ ml/minute} \times 60 \text{ minutes} = 12 \text{ ml/hr}$$

$$\frac{5 \text{ mU/minute}}{10 \text{ mU/ml}} = 0.5 \text{ ml/minute} \times 60 \text{ minutes} = 30 \text{ ml/hr}$$

3. Titration factor (see Chapter 8): To increase the concentration by increments of 1 mU/minute, the hourly rate on the volumetric pump must increase by 6 ml/hr (see above infusion rate). The titration factor for this problem is 6 ml/hr. To increase the concentration to a higher rate, multiply the rate of increase times 6 ml/hr. (Example: Increase infusion to 5 mU/min, multiply 5×6 ml = 30 ml/hr.)

In summary, the secondary IV line, the concentration of the solution is 10 mU/ml of oxytocin with the infusion rate of 30 ml/hr to be increased in increments of 6 ml to 12 ml every 10 minutes until contractions are 2 to 3 minutes apart.

Primary IV

The secondary IV rate will start at 30 ml/hr; therefore, the primary rate will be 70 ml/hr. (Recall that a balance is needed to achieve 100 ml/hr.)

Drop rate using a 10 gtts/ml set is

$$\frac{70 \text{ ml/hr} \times 10 \text{ gtts/ml}}{60 \text{ minutes}} = 11.6 \text{ or } 12 \text{ gtts/min}$$

For every increase in rate from the secondary line, a corresponding decrease must be made with the primary IV line. If the rate of the secondary line exceeds the ordered hourly rate, the primary IV may be shut off completely. The concentration of the solution may be changed by the physician if the mother is receiving too much fluid.

Administration by Volume

In the previous example, the oxytocin was ordered to infuse by concentration, mU/min, which is the recommended method for patient safety. Sometimes in clinical practice, the infusion rate may be ordered by volume, ml/hr.

EXAMPLE

1. Mix 10 units of oxytocin in 1000 NS. Start at 30 ml/hr, increase by 6 to 12 ml q 10 min until uterine contractions are 2 to 3 minutes apart, not to exceed 40 mU/minute.

To determine the concentration per hour of infusion, multiply concentration of the solution $\times$ volume/hr = concentration/hr:

$$10 \text{ mU/ml} \times 30 \text{ ml/hr} = 300 \text{ mU/hr}$$

To determine the concentration of the infusion per minute, divide:

$$\frac{\text{concentration/hour}}{60 \text{ minutes/hour}} = \text{concentration/minute}$$

$$\frac{300 \text{ mU/hr}}{60 \text{ min/hr}} = 5 \text{ mU/minute}$$

Therefore, the oxytocin solution with a concentration of 10 mU/ml at 30 ml/hr will administer 5 mU/minute.

INTRAVENOUS LOADING DOSES

Some situations require intravenous medications to be infused over a short period of time to obtain a serum level for a therapeutic effect. This type of IV drug administration is called a loading dose.

In the following example, a preeclampsia patient receives a loading dose of magnesium sulfate, followed by a maintenance dose of magnesium sulfate, via the secondary IV line. A primary IV line is also maintained after the loading dose is given. At the end of this example, the total IV intake is determined for an 8 hour period.

EXAMPLE

1. Mix magnesium sulfate 20 g in 1000 ml D_5W.
2. Infuse 4 g over 20 minutes, then maintain at 1 g/hr.
3. D_5 LRS at 75 ml/hr, start after magnesium sulfate loading dose.

Available: Secondary Set:
                Magnesium sulfate 50% (5 g in 10 ml ampules)
                1000 ml D_5W
                Microdrip IV set 60 gtts/ml
                Volumetric pump

Primary Set:
1000 ml D_5 LRS
IV set drop factor 10 gtts/ml

For the *secondary* IV, the following calculations must be made:

1. Calculate dose of magnesium sulfate in IV.
2. Concentration of solution.
3. Volume of loading dose and flow rate for volumetric pump (Chapter 6).
4. Infusion rate: volume/hour of magnesium sulfate infusion.

For the *primary* IV, the following calculation must be made:

1. Drop rate/minute.

For the total IV intake, the following solutions must be added:

1. Volume of loading dose.
2. Volume of secondary IV for 8 hours.
3. Volume of primary IV for 8 hours.

Secondary IV

1. $\dfrac{D}{H} \times V = \dfrac{20\ g}{5\ g} \times 10\ ml = 40\ ml$ of magnesium sulfate or 4 ampules

2. Concentration of solution

$$20\ g = 20{,}000\ mg$$
$$20{,}000\ mg \ : \ 1000\ ml \ :: \ X \ : \ 1\ ml$$
$$1000\ X = 20{,}000$$
$$X = 20\ mg$$

The concentration of solution is 20 mg/ml.

3. Volume of loading dose   Flow rate for volumetric pump

$$4\ g = 4000\ mg$$
$$20\ mg \ : \ 1\ ml \ :: \ 4000\ mg \ : \ X \qquad 200\ ml \div \dfrac{20\ min}{60\ min/hr} =$$
$$20\ X = 4000$$
$$X = 200\ ml$$

$$200 \times \dfrac{\overset{3}{\cancel{60}}}{\underset{1}{\cancel{20}}} = 600\ ml/hr$$

The rate on the volumetric pump for the 4 g infusion of magnesium sulfate over 20 minutes will be 600 ml/hr. If the pump cannot be adjusted to that rate, then the infusion rate must be monitored closely and the patient observed for response to drug therapy.

4. Infusion rate: volume/hour

$$1 \text{ g} = 1000 \text{ mg}$$

$$\frac{\text{concentration/hr}}{\text{concentration of sol.}} = \text{volume/hr} \qquad \frac{1000 \text{ mg/hr}}{20 \text{ mg/ml}} = 50 \text{ ml/hr}$$

The rate on the volumetric pump for the 1 g/hr infusion will be 50 ml/hr.

Primary IV

After the loading dose of magnesium sulfate, the primary IV will run at 75 ml/hr.

Drop rate using a 10 gtts/ml set is

$$\frac{75 \text{ ml/hr} \times 10 \text{ gtts/min}}{60 \text{ minutes}} = 12.5 \text{ or } 13 \text{ gtts/min}$$

Total IV intake over 8 hours:

Volume of loading dose		200 ml
Volume of secondary IV	50 ml × 8 =	400 ml
Volume of primary IV	75 ml × 8 =	600 ml
		1200 ml

Since fluid overload is a potential problem for preeclampsia patients, all IV fluids must be calculated accurately.

INTRAVENOUS FLUID BOLUS

An IV fluid bolus is a large volume of 200 to 500 ml of IV fluid infused over a short period of time, one hour or less. A bolus may be given prior to conductive anesthesia or to a preterm patient in labor.

For the next example, calculate the flow rate of an IV bolus from the primary IV, followed by an infusion of a tocolytic drug given by titration. At the end of this example, calculate the patient's fluid intake for 8 hours.

EXAMPLE

1. Start 1000 D_5 LRS at 300 ml × 10 minutes, then reduce to 125 ml/hr.
2. Mix terbutaline 5 mg in 1000 ml NS, start at 10 mcg/min, increase 5 mcg/min q 10 minutes until contractions subside.

Available: Primary set:

  1000 ml D_5 LRS

  IV set drop factor 10 gtts/ml

  Secondary set:

  Terbutaline 1 mg/ml

  500 ml NSS

  Microdrip IV set 60 gtts/ml

  Volumetric pump

For the *secondary* IV, the following calculations must be made:

1. Calculate the dose of terbutaline in IV.
2. Concentration of solution.
3. Infusion rates: volume/minute and hour.
4. Titration factor for 5 mcg/ml.

For the *primary* IV, determine the following:

1. Drop rate/minute for 300 ml over 10 minutes and 125 ml/hr.
2. Balance the primary IV with the secondary IV to achieve a rate of 125 ml/hr.

Total the IV fluids for 8 hours.

Secondary IV

1. $\dfrac{D}{H} \times V = \dfrac{5 \text{ mg}}{1 \text{ mg}} \times 1 \text{ ml} = 5$ ml of terbutaline or 5 ampules

2. Concentration of solution

$$5 \text{ mg} = 5000 \text{ mcg}$$
$$5000 \text{ mcg} \;:\; 1000 \text{ ml} \;::\; X \;:\; 1 \text{ ml}$$
$$1000 \text{ X} = 5000$$
$$X = 5 \text{ mcg}$$

The concentration of solution is 5 mcg/ml.

3. Infusion rates: volume/minute and hour

$$\frac{10 \text{ mcg/min}}{5 \text{ mcg/ml}} = 2 \text{ ml/min} \times 60 \text{ min/hr} = 120 \text{ ml/hr}$$

4. Titration factor: To increase the concentration by increments of 5 mcg/min, the volume of the increment of change must be calculated per minute and hour:

$$\frac{\text{concentration/minute}}{\text{concentration of sol.}} = \text{ml/min} \qquad \frac{5 \text{ mcg/min}}{5 \text{ mcg/ml}} = 1 \text{ ml/min}$$

$$\text{volume/min} \times 60 \text{ min/hr} = \text{volume/hr}$$
$$1 \text{ ml/min} \times 60 \text{ min/hr} = 60 \text{ ml/hr}$$

The titration factor is 1 ml/min or 60 ml/hr. Increasing or decreasing the infusion rate by 5 mcg/min will correspond to an increase or decrease in volume by 1 ml/min or 60 ml/hr.

Primary IV

1. Drop rate for 300 ml over 10 minutes

$$\frac{300 \text{ ml} \times 10 \text{ gtts/ml}}{10 \text{ minutes}} = 300 \text{ gtts/min} \qquad \begin{array}{l} \text{Since this rate is too fast to} \\ \text{count, the flow must be} \\ \text{monitored closely.} \end{array}$$

Drop rate for 125 ml/hr

$$\frac{125 \text{ ml} \times 10 \text{ gtts/ml}}{60 \text{ minutes}} = 20.8 \text{ or } 21 \text{ gtts/min}$$

Total IV intake over 8 hours:

Volume of loading dose		300 ml
Volume of primary set	125 ml × 8 =	1000 ml
Volume of secondary set	180 ml × 8 =	1440 ml
(Assume an average		2740 ml
180 ml/hr was given)		

SUMMARY PRACTICE PROBLEMS

1. Preterm labor.

   a. Give NS 500 ml over 15 minutes, then infuse at 100 ml/hr.

   b. If contractions are still regular, mix ritodrine 150 mg in 500 cc NS. Infuse at 50 mcg/minute and increase by 50 mcg q 10 minutes until contractions cease. Do not infuse more than 350 mcg/min.

Available: Primary set:

1000 ml NS

IV set with drop factor of 10 gtts/ml

Secondary set:

Ritodrine 50 mg in 5 ml ampules

500 ml NS

Microdrip set 60 gtts/ml

Volumetric pump

Determine the following:

a. Secondary IV:

(1) Ritodrine dosage.

(2) Concentration of solution.

(3) Infusion rate for
volume/minute and hour.

(4) Titration factor.

b. Primary IV:

(1) Drop rate for 500 ml over
15 minutes and 100 ml/hr.

c. Total fluid intake for 8 hours:

ANSWER

a. Secondary IV:

$$(1)\ \frac{D}{H} \times V = \frac{150\ mg}{50\ mg} \times 5\ ml = 15\ ml$$ Add 15 ml of ritodrine or
3 ampules to 500 ml
NS.

(2) Concentration of solution

150 mg : 500 ml :: X : 1 ml

500 X = 150

X = 0.3 mg/ml

or

300 mcg/ml

(3) Infusion rates: volume/minute and hour

$$\frac{50 \text{ mcg/min}}{300 \text{ mcg/ml}} = 0.16 \text{ ml/min} \times 60 \text{ min/hr} = 9.6$$

or

10 ml/hr

(4) Titration factor: Since the increment of increase is 50 mcg/minute, the volume/hour, 10 ml/hr, is the titration factor, which increases the concentration by 50 mcg.

b. Primary IV:

(1) Drop rate for 500 ml over 15 minutes

$$\frac{500 \text{ ml} \times 10 \text{ gtts/ml}}{15 \text{ minutes}} = 333 \text{ gtts/min}$$

This rate is impossible to count. Therefore, the infusion must be monitored closely during infusion time.

Drop rate for 100 ml/hr

$$\frac{100 \text{ ml} \times 10 \text{ gtts/ml}}{60 \text{ minutes}} = 16.6 \text{ or } 17 \text{ gtts/ml}$$

c. Total IV intake for 8 hours:

IV fluid bolus	500 ml
Primary IV 100 ml × 8 hr	800 ml
Secondary IV 50 ml × 8 hr	400 ml
(Assume an average of 50 ml/hr)	1700 ml

2. Preeclamptic labor.

a. Mix magnesium sulfate 20 g in 1000 D_5W.

b. Infuse 4 g over 30 minutes, then maintain at 2 g/hr.

c. Lactated Ringer's 1000 ml at 50 ml/hr, start after loading dose of magnesium sulfate.

Available: Secondary set:

              Magnesium sulfate 50% (5 g in 10 ml)

              D_5W 1000 ml

              Microdrop IV set 60 gtts/ml

              Volumetric pump

Primary set:

Lactated Ringer's 1000 ml

IV set 10 gtts/ml

Determine the following:

a. Secondary IV:

(1) Magnesium sulfate dosage.

(2) Concentration of solution.

(3) Volume of loading dose and infusion rate for volumetric pump.

(4) Infusion rate per hour of magnesium sulfate.

b. Primary IV:

(1) Drop rate for 50 ml/hr.

c. Total fluid intake for 8 hours:

ANSWER

a. Secondary IV:

(1) $\dfrac{D}{H} \times V = \dfrac{20\ g}{5\ g} \times 10\ ml = 40\ ml$ of magnesium sulfate or 4 ampules

(2) 20 g = 20,000 mg

$$20{,}000\ mg \quad : \quad 1000\ ml \quad :: \quad X\ mg \quad : \quad 1\ ml$$
$$1000\ X = 20{,}000$$
$$X = 20\ mg$$

The concentration of solution is 20 mg/ml.

(3) Volume of loading dose

4 g = 4000 mg

$$20\ mg : 1\ ml :: 4000\ mg : X\ ml$$
$$20\ X = 4000$$
$$X = 200\ ml$$

Infusion rate for 30 minutes

$$200\ ml \div \dfrac{30\ min}{60\ min/hr} =$$

$$200 \times \dfrac{\overset{2}{\cancel{60}}}{\underset{1}{\cancel{30}}} = 400\ ml/hr$$

(4) Infusion rate: volume/hour

2 g = 2000 mg

$$\dfrac{2000\ mg/hr}{20\ mg/ml} = 100\ ml/hr$$

b. Primary IV:

(1) After the loading dose

$$\frac{50 \text{ ml/hr} \times 10 \text{ gtts/min}}{60 \text{ minutes}} = 8.3 \text{ or } 8 \text{ gtts/min}$$

c. Total IV intake over 8 hours:

Volume of loading dose		200 ml
Volume of secondary IV	100 ml × 8 =	800 ml
Volume of primary IV	50 ml × 8 =	400 ml
		1400 ml

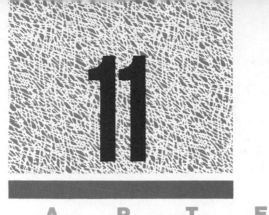

11

C H A P T E R

Community

- Identify the problems with conversion of metric to household measure.
- Name the components of a solution.
- List three methods for preparing a solution.
- Recognize three ways solutions are labeled.
- State the formula used for calculating a solution of a desired concentration.
- State the formula used for calculating a weaker solution from a stronger solution.

Although the metric system has become widespread in the clinical area, the home setting generally does not have the devices of metric measure. This becomes a problem when liquid medication is prescribed in metric measure for the home patient. The community nurse should be able to assist the client in converting metric to household when necessary.

Preparation of solutions in the home setting may involve conversion between the metric and household systems. Solutions used in the home setting can be used for oral fluid replacement, topical application, irrigations, or disinfectants. Although the majority of the solutions are commercially available, solutions that can be prepared in the home can be effective and less costly than the premixed items.

When commercially prepared drugs are too concentrated for the client's use and must be diluted, it becomes necessary to calculate the strength of the solution to meet the therapeutic need as prescribed by the physician. Knowledge of solution preparation and metric-household conversion can be a useful skill for the community nurse.

METRIC TO HOUSEHOLD CONVERSION

When changing from metric to household measure, the ounce from the apothecary system is used as an intermediary because there is no clear conversion between the two systems.

The conversion factors for volume are:

ounces to milliliters, multiply ounces times 29.57

milliliters to ounces, multiply milliliters times 0.034

The conversion factors for weight are:

ounces to grams, multiply ounces times 28.35

grams to ounces, multiply grams times 0.035

Note that weight and volume measures differ in the metric system. The properties of crystals, powders, and other solids account for the differences more so than do liquids. Also, as liquid measures increase in volume, there are further discrepancies between metric and standard household measure. Table 11–1 shows the current approximate equivalents. Deciliters and liters are also included with volume measurements. These terms will be seen more frequently as the use of the metric system increases. Although conversion charts are helpful guides, a metric measuring device would be optimal for drug administration. Standard household measuring devices should be used instead of tableware if a metric device is not available.

TABLE 11-1 Household to Metric Conversions _____

Standard Household Measure	Apothecary	Metric Volume	Metric Weight
⅛ teaspoon (t)	7–8 gtts/¹⁄₄₈ oz	0.6 ml	0.6 g
¼ teaspoon	15 gtts/¹⁄₂₄ oz	1.25 ml	1.25 g
½ teaspoon	30 gtts/¹⁄₁₂ oz	2.5 ml	2.5 g
1 teaspoon	60 gtts/⅙ oz	5 ml	5 g
1 tablespoon (T)/ 3 teaspoons	½ oz	15 ml	15 g
2 tablespoons/ 6 teaspoons	1 oz	¼ dl/30 ml	30 g
¼ cup/4 tablespoons	2 oz	½ dl/60 ml	55 g
⅓ cup/5 tablespoons	2½ oz	¾ dl/75 ml	75 g
½ cup	4 oz	1 dl/120 ml	110 g
1 cup	8 oz	¼ L/240–250 ml	225 g
1 pint	16 oz	½ L/480–500 ml	
1 quart	32 oz	1 L/1000 ml	
2 quarts/½ gallon	64 oz	2 L/2000 ml	
1 gallon	128 oz	3¾ L/3840–4000 ml	

Practice Problems

Use Table 11-1 to convert metric to household.

1. Dimetapp 2.5 ml every 6 hours as necessary.

_____

2. Ceclor 5 ml 4 times a day.

_____

3. Tylenol elixir 1.25 ml every 6 hours as necessary for temperature greater than 102°F.

_____

4. Maalox 30 ml after meals and at bedtime.

_____

5. Neo-Calglucon 7.5 ml 3 times a day.

_____

6. Basaljel 45 ml after each meal.

_____

7. Castor oil 60 ml at bedtime.

_____

8. Metamucil 5 g in one glass of water every morning.

_____

9. Dilantin-30 suspension 10 ml twice a day.

---

10. Homemade pediatric electrolyte solution.

H_2O 1 liter, boiled
sugar 30 g
salt 1.5 g
lite salt 2.5 g
baking soda 2.5 g

ANSWERS

1. Dimetapp 2.5 ml = ½ t
2. Ceclor 5 ml = 1 t
3. Tylenol elixir 1.25 ml = ¼ t
4. Maalox 30 ml = 2 T
5. Neo-Calglucon 7.5 ml = 1½ t
6. Basaljel 45 ml = 3 T
7. Castor oil 60 ml = 4 T or ¼ c
8. Metamucil 5 g = 1 t
9. Dilantin-30 suspension 10 ml = 2 t
10. H_2O 1 liter = 1 qt
    sugar 30 g = 2 T
    salt 1.25 g = ¼ t
    lite salt 2.5 g = ½ t
    baking soda 2.5 g = ½ t

PREPARING A SOLUTION OF A DESIRED CONCENTRATION

All solutions contain a solute (drug) and a solvent (liquid). Solutions can be mixed three different ways:

1. *Weight to Weight:* Involves mixing the weight of a given solute with the weight of a given liquid.

Example: 5 g sugar with 100 g H_2O

This type of preparation is used in the pharmaceutical setting and is the *most accurate.* Scales for weight to weight preparation are not usually found in the home setting.

2. *Weight to Volume:* Uses the weight of a given solute with the volume of an appropriate amount of solvent.

Example: 10 g of salt in 1 L of H_2O

or

2 oz of salt in 1 qt of H_2O

Again, a scale is needed for this preparation.

3. *Volume to Volume:* Means a given volume of solution is mixed with a given volume of solution.

Example: 10 ml of hydrogen peroxide 3% in 1 dl H_2O

or

2 T of hydrogen peroxide 3% in ½ c H_2O

Preparing solutions volume to volume is commonly used in both the clinical and home setting.

After a solution is prepared, the strength can be expressed numerically three different ways:

1. A ratio—1:20 acetic acid

2. A fraction—5 g/100 ml acetic acid

3. A percentage—5% acetic acid

With a ratio, the first number is the solute and the second number is the solvent. In a fraction, the numerator is the drug and the denominator is the liquid. A solution labeled by percentage indicates the amount of solute in 100 ml of liquid. All pharmaceutically prepared solutions use the metric system, and the ratio, fraction, and percentages are interpreted in *gram/milliliter*.

Changing a Ratio to Fractions and Percentage

A ratio can be changed to a percentage or a fraction by setting up a proportion using the following variables:

known drug : known volume = desired drug : desired volume

A proportion can also be set up like a fraction:

$$\frac{\text{known drug}}{\text{known volume}} = \frac{\text{desired drug}}{\text{desired volume}}$$

Remember: Any variable in this formula can be found if the other three variables are known.

EXAMPLE

Problem 1:   Change acetic acid 1:20 to a percentage

$$1 \text{ g} : 20 \text{ ml} = X \text{ g} : 100 \text{ ml}$$
$$20 X = 100$$
$$X = 5 \text{ g}$$

$$1 \text{ g} : 20 \text{ ml} = 5 \text{ g} : 100 \text{ ml}$$

NOTE: In percentage, the volume of liquid is 100 ml.

The ratio can be expressed as a fraction, 5 g/100 ml, or as a percentage, 5%. Another method of changing a ratio to a percentage involves finding a multiple of 100 for volume (denominator), then multiplying both terms by that multiple.

Practice Problems

Change the following ratios to fractions and percentages.

1. 4:1

2. 2:1

3. 1:50

4. 1:3

5. 1:1000

6. 1:10,000

7. 1:4

8. 1:5000

9. 1:200

10. 1:10

ANSWERS

1. $4 : 1 = X : 100$
$X = 400$

$\dfrac{400}{100}$, 400%

2. $2 : 1 = X : 100$
$X = 200$

$\dfrac{200}{100}$, 200%

3. $1 : 50 = X : 100$
$50 X = 100$
$X = 2$

$\dfrac{2}{100}$, 2%

4. $1 : 3 = X : 100$
$3 X = 100$
$X = 33.3$

$\dfrac{33.3}{100}$, 33.3%

5. $1 : 1000 = X : 100$
$1000 X = 100$
$X = 0.1$

$\dfrac{0.1}{100}$, 0.1%

6. $1 : 10,000 = X : 100$
$10,000 X = 100$
$X = 0.01$

$\dfrac{1}{10,000}$, 0.01%

7. $1 : 4 = X : 100$
$4 X = 100$
$X = 25$

$\dfrac{25}{100}$, 25%

8. $1 : 5000 = X : 100$
$5000 X = 100$
$X = 0.02$

$\dfrac{0.02}{100}$, 0.02%

9. $1 : 200 = X : 100$
$200 X = 100$
$X = 0.5$

$\dfrac{0.5}{100}$, 0.5%

10. $1 : 10 = X : 100$

$\quad 10\,X = 100$

$X = 10$

$$\frac{10}{100},\ 10\%$$

In the previous problems, gm/ml was the unit of measure used for preparing solutions. Scales for measuring grams are rarely found in the clinical area or the home environment. Volume (ml) is the common measurement of drugs for administration. Drugs that are powders, crystals, and liquids are measured in graduated measuring cups with metric, apothecary, or household measure. The milliliter, although a volume measure, can be substituted for a gram, a measure of mass, because at 4°C, 1 milliliter of water weighs 1 gram. Mass and volume differ with the type of substance, thus grams and milliliters are not exact equivalents in all instances, but they can be accepted as approximate values for solution preparation.

Calculating a Solution From a Ratio

To obtain a solution from a ratio, use the proportion or fraction method.

EXAMPLES

Problem 1: Prepare 500 ml of a 1:100 vinegar-water solution for a vaginal douche.

known drug : known volume : : desired drug : desired volume

$1\ ml:100\ ml=X\ ml:500\ ml$

$100\,X = 500$

$X = 5\ ml$

or

$$\frac{\text{known drug}}{\text{known volume}} = \frac{\text{desired drug}}{\text{desired volume}}$$

$$\frac{1\ ml}{100\ ml} = \frac{X}{500\ ml}$$

$$100\,X = 500$$

$$X = 5\ ml$$

Answer: 5 ml of vinegar added to 500 ml of water is a 1:100 vinegar solution.

NOTE: 5 ml did not increase the volume of the solution by a large amount. When mixing volume and volume solutions, the total amount of *desired volume* should not be exceeded. Therefore, it is important to determine the volume of desired drug first, then remove that volume from the appropriate amount of solvent (solution). When mixing the solution, add the desired drug first, then follow with the premeasured solvent. This process will make the solution have an accurate concentration.

Problem 2: Prepare 100 ml of a 1:4 hydrogen peroxide 3% and normal saline mouthwash.

known drug : known volume : : desired drug : desired volume
$$1 \text{ ml} \quad : \quad 4 \text{ ml} \quad = \quad X \quad : \quad 100 \text{ ml}$$
$$4 X = 100 \text{ ml}$$
$$X = 25 \text{ ml}$$

25 ml of hydrogen peroxide 3% is the amount of desired drug. To calculate the amount of normal saline, use the following formula:

desired volume − desired drug = desired solvent
$$100 \text{ ml} \quad - \quad 25 \text{ ml} \quad = \quad 75 \text{ ml}$$

Answer: 75 ml of saline and 25 ml of hydrogen peroxide 3% make a 1:4 mouthwash.

Calculating a Solution from a Percentage

To obtain a solution from a percentage, use the same formula with either the proportion or fraction method.

EXAMPLE

Problem 1: Prepare 1000 ml of a 0.9% NaCl solution.

known drug : known volume : : desired drug : desired volume
$$0.9 \text{ g} \quad : \quad 100 \text{ ml} \quad = \quad X \quad : \quad 1000 \text{ ml}$$
$$100 X = 900$$
$$X = 9 \text{ g}$$

or

9 ml

Answer: 9 g or 9 ml of NaCl in 1000 ml will make a 0.9% NaCl solution.

PREPARING A WEAKER SOLUTION FROM A STRONGER SOLUTION

When a situation requires the preparation of a weaker solution from a stronger solution, the amount of desired drug must again be determined. The known variables are the desired solution, the available or on hand solution, and the desired volume. The formula can be set up with the strength of the solutions expressed in either ratio or percentage. The proportion method or the fractional method can be used to solve the problem. The first ratio or fraction, being the desired solution (weaker solution), is the numerator, and the available or on hand solution (stronger solution) is the denominator.

desired solution : available solution : : desired drug : desired volume

or

$$\frac{\text{desired solution}}{\text{available solution}} = \frac{\text{desired drug}}{\text{desired volume}}$$

EXAMPLE

Problem 1: Prepare 500 ml of a 2.5% aluminum acetate solution from a 5% aluminum acetate solution. Use water as the solvent.

$$2.5\% \,:\, 5\% \,= X : 500 \text{ ml}$$
$$2.5 \text{ ml} : 5 \text{ ml} = X : 500 \text{ ml}$$
$$5\,X = 1250$$
$$X = 250 \text{ ml}$$

Answer: Use 250 ml of 5% aluminum acetate to make the 500 ml of 2.5% aluminum acetate solution.

Determine the amount of water needed.

desired volume − desired drug = desired solvent
500 ml   −   250 ml   =   250 ml

or

Same problem using the fraction method.

$$\frac{2.5\%}{5\%} \times \frac{X}{500 \text{ ml}} =$$
$$5X = 1250$$
$$X = 250 \text{ ml of 5\% aluminum acetate}$$

or

Same problem but stated as a ratio.

Prepare 500 ml of a 1:40 aluminum acetate solution from a 1:20 aluminum acetate solution with water as the solvent.

$$\frac{1}{40} : \frac{1}{20} = \text{ X} : 500 \text{ ml}$$

$$\frac{1}{20 \text{ X}} = \frac{500}{40}$$

$$\text{X} = \frac{500}{\underset{2}{\cancel{40}}} \times \frac{\overset{1}{\cancel{20}}}{1} = \frac{500}{2}$$

$$\text{X} = 250 \text{ ml of 5\% aluminum acetate solution}$$

GUIDELINES FOR HOME SOLUTIONS

For solutions prepared by clients in the home, the directions need to be very specific and written if possible. People often think more is better. Teach the client the dangers of the solutions if they are too concentrated. Higher concentrations of solutions can be irritating to tissues and prevent the desired effect. Recommend that standard measuring spoons and cups be used rather than tableware. Level measures rather than heaping measures of dry solutes should be used. Utensils and containers for solution preparation should be *clean or sterilized by boiling* if used for infants. Avoid mixing acidic solutions in aluminum containers, especially if the solution is for oral use. Although there is no evidence of toxicity, a metallic taste will be noticeable. Glass, enamel, or plastic may be substituted. Solutions should be made fresh daily or prior to use. Oral solutions, especially for infants, need refrigeration, but it is not necessary for topical solutions.

When preparing the solution, add the desired drug first, then the solvent. This helps to disperse the solute and ensures that the desired volume of solution is not exceeded.

Solution problems are best calculated within the metric system. Fractional and percentage dosages are difficult to determine within the household system.

SUMMARY PRACTICE PROBLEMS

Identify the known variables and choose the appropriate formula. Calculate the following solutions using the metric system. Use the conversion table to obtain the household equivalent.

1. Prepare 250 ml of a 0.6% NaCl and sterile water solution for nose drops.

   _____

2. Prepare 250 ml of a 5% glucose and sterile water solution for an infant feeding.

   _____

3. Prepare 1000 ml of a 25% Betadine solution with sterile saline for a foot soak.

   _____

4. Prepare 2 L of a 2% Lysol solution for cleaning a changing area.

   _____

5. Prepare 20 L of a 2% sodium bicarbonate solution for a bath.

   _____

6. Prepare 100 ml of a 50% hydrogen peroxide 3% and water mouthwash.

   _____

7. Prepare 500 ml of a modified Dakin's solution 0.5% from a 5% sodium hypochlorite solution with sterile water as the solvent.

   _____

8. Prepare 1500 ml of a 0.9% NaCl solution for an enema.

   _____

9. Prepare 2 L of a 1:1000 Neosporin bladder irrigation with sterile saline. Omit the household conversion.

   _____

10. Determine how much alcohol is needed in a 3:1 alcohol and white vinegar solution for an external ear irrigation. 30 ml of vinegar is used. Solve with the proportion method.

   _____

11. Prepare 1000 ml of a 1:10 sodium hypochlorite and water solution for cleaning.

   _____

12. Prepare 1000 ml of a 3% sodium hypochlorite and water solution.

   _____

ANSWERS

1. Known drug   0.6% NaCl $0.6 : 100 = X : 250$

    Known volume   100 ml $100 X = 150$

    Desired drug   X $X = 1.5$ ml

    Desired volume   250 ml

1.5 ml of NaCl in 250 ml of water will yield a 0.6% NaCl solution. Household equivalents will be approximately ¼ teaspoon NaCl and 1 cup sterile water.

2. Known drug   5% glucose (sugar) $5 : 100 = X : 250$

    Known volume   100 ml $100 X = 1250$

    Desired drug   X $X = 12.5$ ml

    Desired volume   250 ml

12.5 ml of sugar in 250 ml of water will yield a 5% glucose solution. Household equivalents will be approximately 1 tablespoon in 1 cup of sterile water.

3. Known drug   25% Betadine $25 : 100 = X : 1000$

    Known volume   100 ml $100 X = 25000$

    Desired drug   X $X = 250$ ml

    Desired volume   1000 ml   1000 ml − 250 ml = 750 ml

250 ml of Betadine in 750 ml saline will yield a 25% Betadine solution. Household equivalents will be 1 cup Betadine in sterile saline.

4. Known drug   2% Lysol $2 : 100 = X : 2000$ ml

    Known volume   100 ml $100 X = 4000$

    Desired drug   X $X = 40$ ml

    Desired volume   2 L = 2000 ml

40 ml of Lysol in 2 L of water will yield a 2% Lysol solution. Household equivalents will be 2 tablespoons and 2 teaspoons (40 ml) of Lysol to 2 quarts or ½ gallon of water.

5. Known drug   2% sodium bicarbonate $2 : 100 = X : 20,000$ ml

    Known volume   100 ml $100 X = 40,000$

    Desired drug   X $X = 400$ ml or

    Desired volume   20,000 ml   400 g

400 ml or 400 g of sodium bicarbonate (baking soda) in 20,000 ml will yield a 2% sodium bicarbonate solution. Household equivalents will be 1 ½ cups and 2 tablespoons baking soda in 5 gallons of water.

6. Known drug   50% hydrogen peroxide $50 : 100 = X : 100$

    Known volume   100 ml $100 X = 5000$

    Desired drug   X $X = 50$ ml

    Desired volume   100 ml   100 ml − 50 ml = 50 ml

50 ml of hydrogen peroxide 3% with 50 ml water will yield a 50% solution. Household equivalents will be approximately 3 tablespoons of hydrogen peroxide in 3 tablespoons of water.

7. Desired solution   0.5% $0.5 : 5 = X : 500$

  Available $5 X = 250$
    solution   5% $X = 50$ ml
  Desired drug   X 500 ml $- 50$ ml $= 450$ ml
  Desired volume   500 ml

50 ml of sodium hypochlorite with 450 ml sterile water will yield a 0.5% modified Dakin's solution. Household equivalents will be 3 tablespoons and 1 teaspoon to 1 pint minus 3 tablespoons of water.

8. Known drug   0.9% $0.9 : 100 = X : 1500$

  Known volume   100 ml $100 X = 1350$
  Desired drug   X $X = 13.5$ ml
  Desired volume   1500 ml

13.5 ml of NaCl with 1500 ml water will yield a 0.9% NaCl solution. Household equivalents will be 1½ quarts of water and 2½ teaspoons of salt.

9. Known drug   1 ml $1 : 1000 = X : 2000$

  Known volume   1000 ml $1000 X = 2000$
  Desired drug   X $X = 2$ ml
  Desired volume   2000 ml

2 ml of Neosporin irrigant added to 2000 ml sterile saline will yield a 1:1000 solution for a continuous bladder irrigation. This treatment is done primarily in the clinical setting.

10. Use a ratio and proportion to solve this problem.

$$3 : 1 : : X : 30 \text{ ml}$$
$$X = 90 \text{ ml}$$

Add 90 ml of alcohol to 30 ml of vinegar to yield a 3:1 solution for an external ear wash. Household equivalents will be 6 tablespoons of alcohol with 2 tablespoons of vinegar.

11. Known drug   1 ml $1 : 10 : : X : 1000$

  Known volume   10 ml $10 X = 1000$
  Desired drug   X $X = 100$ ml
  Desired volume   1000 ml 1000 ml $- 100$ ml $= 900$ ml

100 ml of sodium hypochlorite (bleach) in 900 ml water will yield a 1:10 sodium hypochlorite solution. Household equivalents will be ⅓ cup and 2 tablespoons in approximately 1 quart water minus ⅓ cup and 2 tablespoons of water.

12. Known drug   3 ml   3 : 100 : : X : 1000

Known volume   100 ml   100 X = 3000

Desired drug   X   X = 30 ml

Desired volume   1000 ml   1000 ml − 30 ml = 970 ml

30 ml of sodium hypochlorite (bleach) in 970 ml water will yield a 3% sodium hypochlorite solution. Household equivalents will be 2 tablespoons in 1 quart water minus 2 tablespoons of water.

REFERENCES

Abrams, A.: Clinical Drug Therapy. Philadelphia, J. B. Lippincott Co., 1983.

Arcangelo, V. P., Weaver, M. E., and Koehler, V. J.: Programmed Mathematics of Drugs and Solutions. Philadelphia, J. B. Lippincott Co., 1984.

Aurigemma, A., and Bohny, B.: Dosage Calculation, 2nd ed. New York, National League for Nursing, 1984.

Axton, S. E., and Fugate, T.: A Protocol for Pediatric IV Meds. American Journal of Nursing, 87, 7:943–945, July 1987.

Behrman, R. E., and Vaughan, V. C.: Nelson Textbook of Pediatrics, 12th ed. Philadelphia, W. B. Saunders Co., 1983.

Biller, J., and Yeager, A. (eds.): The Harriet Lane Handbook, 9th ed. Chicago, Year Book Medical Publishers, Inc., 1981.

Blume, D. M., and Cornett, E. F.: Dosages and Solutions, 4th ed. Philadelphia, F.A. Davis Co., 1984.

Carey, B.: Microdrop calculations for neonates in converting micrograms/kilograms/minute to microdrops. Dimensions of Critical Care Nursing, 1, 6:338–339, November/December 1982.

Comer, J.: Pharmacology in Critical Care. Bethany, CT, Fleschner Publishing Co., 1981.

Cordon, M.: Clinical Calculations for Nurses. New Jersey, Prentice-Hall, Inc., 1984.

Curren, A. M., and Mundy, L. D.: Math for Meds, 5th ed. San Diego, CA, Wallcur, Inc., 1986.

DeAngelis, R., and Brott, W.: The "factor 15" method in converting micrograms/kilograms/minute to microdrops. Dimensions of Critical Care Nursing, 1, 6:334–337, November/December 1982.

Gilman, A. G., Goodman, L. S., and Gilman, A. (eds.): Goodman and Gilman's The Pharmacological Basis of Therapeutics, 6th ed. New York, Macmillan Co., 1980.

Govoni, L. E., and Hayes, J. E.: Drugs and Nursing Implications, 5th ed. Norwalk, CT, Appleton-Century-Crofts, 1985.

Hegstad, L. N., and Hayek, W.: Essential Drug Dosage Calculations. Bowie, MD, Robert J. Brady Co., 1983.

Howry, L. B., Bindler, R. M., and Tso, Y.: Pediatric Medications. Philadelphia, J.B. Lippincott Co., 1981.

Huey, F.: What's on the market? A nurse's guide. American Journal of Nursing, 83, 6:902–910, 1983.

Intramuscular Injections. Philadelphia, Wyeth Laboratories, 1970.

Johnson, G. G.: Mathematics for Nurses, 2nd ed. Norwalk, CT, Appleton-Century-Crofts, 1986.

Keenan, P.: The "key number" conversion method in converting micrograms/kilograms/minute to microdrops. Dimensions of Critical Care Nursing, 1, 6:332–333, November/December 1982.

Lewis, L. W.: Fundamental Skills in Patient Care, 3rd ed. Philadelphia, J.B. Lippincott Co., 1984.

Loebl, S., and Spratto, G.: The Nurses Drug Handbook, 3rd ed. New York, John Wiley and Sons, 1983.

McGill, S. L., and Smith, J. R.: IV Therapy. Bowie, MD, Robert J. Brady Co., 1981.

Medici, G. A.: Drug Dosage Calculations: A Guide for Current Clinical Practice. New Jersey, Prentice-Hall, Inc., 1980.

Melmon, K., and Morrelli, H. (eds.): Clinical Pharmacology, 2nd ed. New York, Macmillan Co., 1978.

Norville, M. F.: Drug Dosages and Solutions Workbook. Bowie, MD, Robert J. Brady Co., 1982.

Richardson, L. I., and Richardson, J. K.: The Mathematics of Drugs and Solutions with Clinical Applications, 3rd ed. New York, McGraw-Hill Book Co., 1985.

Rosenthal, K.: Charts vs formula method in converting micrograms/kilograms/minute to microdrops. Dimensions of Critical Care Nursing, 1, 6:326–331, November/December 1982.

Russell, H.: Pediatric Drugs and Nursing Interventions. New York, McGraw-Hill Book Co., 1980.

Sackheim G., and Robins L.: Programmed Mathematics, 5th ed. New York, Macmillan Co., 1983.

Scott, M.: Calculations of Medications Using the Proportion. Norwalk, CT, Appleton-Century-Crofts, 1982.

Sheridan, E., Patterson, H. R., and Gustafson, E. A.: Falconer's The Drug, The Nurse, The Patient, 7th ed. Philadelphia, W.B. Saunders Co., 1982.

Vervoren, T. M., and Oppeneer, J. E.: Workbook of Solutions and Dosage of Drugs, 12th ed. St. Louis, C.V. Mosby Co., 1983.

Weyant, H.: Utilization of an intravenous drug guide. Focus on Critical Care, 11, 2:58–62, 1984.

Wiener, M. B., and Pepper, G. A.: Clinical Pharmacology and Therapeutics in Nursing, 2nd ed. New York, McGraw-Hill Book Co., 1985.

Zenk, K. F.: Dosage calculations for drugs administered by infusion. American Journal of Hospital Pharmacy, 37:1304–1305, 1980.

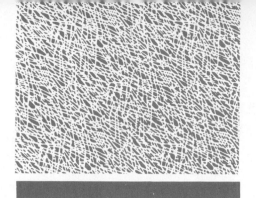

Comprehensive Test

The comprehensive test is for testing content in Part III, oral, inject-able, and intravenous drugs, and in Chapter 7, pediatrics. The test is divided into four sections. There is a total of 25 clinical problems and the test should take an hour or less to complete. You can use the conversion table in Appendix B. Minimum passing score is 80% or 20 correctly an-swered problems. If you have more than two wrong in a section of the test, return to the chapter in the book representing the test section and rework the practice problems.

ORAL PREPARATIONS

1. Order: dipyridamole/Persantine 100 mg, p.o., daily.

Drug available: Persantine 25 mg per tablet.

How many tablets would you give?

2. Order: furosemide/Lasix 20 mg, p.o., bid.
Drug available: Lasix 40 mg scored tablet.
How many tablets would you give?

3. Order: cloxacillin/Tegopen 200 mg, p.o., q8h.
Drug available:

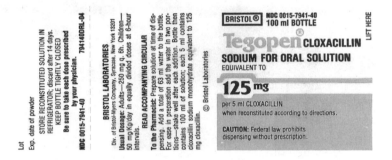

How many ml (cc) would you give?

4. Order: ampicillin/Polycillin 0.5 g, p.o., q12h.
Drug available: ampicillin 250 mg per 5 ml.
How many ml (cc) would you give?
NOTE: Change g to mg before working the problem.

5. Order: acetaminophen/Tylenol gr xv.

Drug available: Tylenol 325 mg per tablet.

How many tablets would you give?

6. Order: morphine gr ⅙, p.o., PRN.

Drug available:

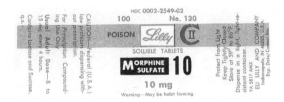

How many tablets would you give?

NOTE: Change gr to mg. See conversion table, Appendix B, if needed.

7. Order: 300 ml of 75% Ensure solution through the nasogastric tube, q6h.

How much Ensure solution and how much water should be mixed to equal 300 ml?

INJECTABLES

8. Order: hydroxyzine/Vistaril 25 mg, deep IM, stat.
Drug available: Vistaril 100 mg/2 ml in a vial.
How many ml would you give?

9. Order: digoxin/Lanoxin 0.25 mg, IM, qd.
Drug available: Lanoxin 0.5 mg/2 ml in an ampule.
How many ml would you give?

10. Order: atropine 0.5 mg, IM, stat.
Drug available:

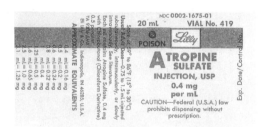

How many ml would you give?

11. Order: meperidine/Demerol 40 mg and atropine SO₄ 0.4 mg, IM, stat.

Drug available: Meperidine 50 mg/ml in prefilled 2 ml cartridge. Atropine SO₄ 0.4 mg/ml in a multiple-dose vial.

How many ml of meperidine and how many ml of atropine would you give?

Explain how the two drugs would be mixed in the cartridge.

12. Order: heparin U 2500, SC, q6h.

Drug available: heparin U 10,000/ml in a multiple-dose (10 ml) vial.

How many ml would you give at each dose?

What type of syringe would you use?

13. Order: cefamandole/Mandol 500 mg, IM, q8h.

Drug available:

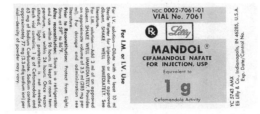

How many ml should be given? (See label for mixing.)

14. Order: penicillin G potassium U 200,000, IM, q6h.

Drug available:

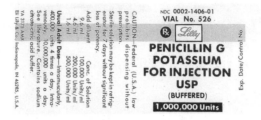

How much diluent will you add to the vial?

How many ml should be given?

INTRAVENOUS

15. Order: 1000 ml of 5% D/½ NSS in 8 hours.

Available: 1 liter of 5% D/½ NSS; IV set labeled 10 gtts/ml.

How many drops per minute should the patient receive?

16. Order: 500 ml of D₅W in 2 hours.

Available: 500 ml of D₅W; IV set labeled 15 gtts/ml.

How many drops per minute should the patient receive?

17. Order: cefamandole/Mandol 600 mg, IV, q6h.

Available: Buretrol set with drop factor 60 gtts/ml; 500 ml D$_5$W.

Drug available:

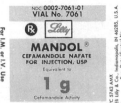

The label reads to dilute with 10 ml for IV use, which yields 10.5 ml of drug solution.

Instruction: dilute drug in 75 ml of D$_5$W and infuse in 30 minutes.

How many gtts/min should the patient receive?

18. Order: cefazolin/Kefzol 500 mg, IV, q6h.

Available: volumetric pump.

Drug available:

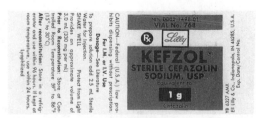

Instruction: dilute in 75 ml and infuse in 30 minutes.

At what rate would you set the volumetric pump?

19. Order: aq. penicillin U 300,000, IV, q4h.

Available: Buretrol set with drop factor of 60 gtts/min; 500 ml D₅W.

Drug available:

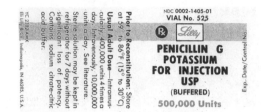

The literature insert reads to add 3.0 ml. The drug solution would equal 3.2 ml.

Instruction: dilute U 300,000 of aq. penicillin in 60 ml of 5% D₅W and infuse 20 minutes.

How many gtts per minute should the patient receive?

PEDIATRICS

20. Child with cardiac disorder.

Order: Lanoxin elixir 0.5 mg, p.o., qd.

Drug available: Lanoxin 0.05 mg/ml.

Child's weight and age: 15 kg, 3 years old.

Pediatric dose: 0.040–0.060 mg/kg.

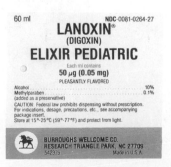

How many ml would you give?

21. Child with fever.

Order: Acetaminophen/Tempra 120 mg, p.o., tid, PRN temp > 102° F.

Drug available: Tempra 160 mg/5 ml.

NDC 0087-0733-04

Do not use if carton overwrap was missing or broken.
For temporary relief of fever, minor aches and pains, and simple headaches due to colds, "flu," chicken pox, other viral infections and immunizations as directed by your physician.
TEMPRA is not likely to cause the occasional side effects associated with the use of aspirin.
Dosage: One dose every 4 hours as needed but not more than 5 times daily.

Age	Dosage
Under 2	As directed by physician
2-3	1 teaspoon
4-5	1½ teaspoons
6-8	2 teaspoons
9-10	2½ teaspoons
11	3 teaspoons
12 & over	3-4 teaspoons

WARNING:
If fever persists for more than 3 days (72 hours) or if pain continues for more than 5 days, consult your physician.
As with any drug, if you are pregnant or nursing a baby, seek the advice of a health professional before using this product.

ACETAMINOPHEN
RELIEVES FEVER
RELIEVES PAIN
ALCOHOL-FREE
CHERRY-FLAVORED SYRUP

4 FL OZ (118 ML)

Each teaspoonful (5 ml) of TEMPRA® syrup contains 160 mg (2.46 grains) of acetaminophen with a delicious, naturally-sweetened cherry flavor (no artificial sweeteners or alcohol used).

Your physician is the best source of counsel and guidance when pain or fever is present.

TEMPRA cherry-flavored drops are available for infants.

KEEP THIS AND ALL MEDICATIONS OUT OF THE REACH OF CHILDREN.

NUTRITIONAL DIVISION
Mead Johnson & Company
Evansville, Indiana 47721 U.S.A.
Made in U.S.A.   ©1983, M.J. & Co.

Child's weight and age: 15 kg, 3 years old.

Pediatric dose: 120–200 mg tid-qid, not to exceed 480 mg/day.

How many ml would you give?

22. Child with strep throat.

Order: penicillin G potassium U 500,000, IM, stat.

Drug available: penicillin G potassium U 500,000/ml.

NDC 0002-1406-01
VIAL No. 526
Ⓡ Lilly
PENICILLIN G POTASSIUM
FOR INJECTION USP
(BUFFERED)
1,000,000 Units

CAUTION—Federal (U.S.A.) law prohibits dispensing without prescription.
Sterile solution may be kept in refrigerator for 7 days without significant loss of potency.

Add diluent	Conc. of Solution
9.6 ml	100,000 Units/ml
4.6 ml	200,000 Units/ml
1.6 ml	500,000 Units/ml

Usual Adult Dose—Intramuscularly, 400,000 units 4 times a day; Intravenously, 10,000,000 units a day. See literature. Contains sodium citrate-citric acid buffer.

TA 3175 AMX
Eli Lilly & Co., Indianapolis, IN 46285, U.S.A.

Exp. Date/Control No.

Child's age: 12 years old.

Pediatric dose: U 300,000–1,200,000 per day.

How many ml would you give?

23. Child with otitis media.

Order: amoxicillin 250 mg, p.o., tid.

Drug available:

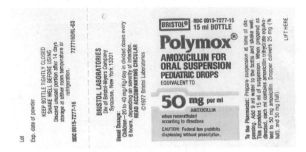

Child's weight and age: 19 kg, 5 years old.

Pediatric dose: 20–40 mg/kg/day in 3 divided doses.

How many ml would you give?

24. Child with asthma.

Order: theophylline elixir 100 mg, p.o., q6h.

Drug available: theophylline elixir 80 mg/15 ml.

Child's weight and age: 22 kg, 7 years old.

Pediatric dose: 400 mg/24 hrs in 4 doses.

How many ml would you give?

25. Child with pruritus.

Order: Benadryl 25 mg, p.o., tid.

Drug available:

N 0071-2220-17

ELIXIR

Benadryl®

(Diphenhydramine
Hydrochloride Elixir, USP)

Caution—Federal law prohibits
dispensing without prescription.

4 FLUIDOUNCES

PARKE-DAVIS
Div of Warner-Lambert Co
Morris Plains, NJ 07950 USA

**Elixir P-D 2220 for prescription
dispensing only.**

Contains—12.5 mg diphenhydramine
hydrochloride in each 5 mL. Alcohol,
14%.

Dose—Adults, 2 to 4 teaspoonfuls; children over 20 lb, 1 to 2 teaspoonfuls;
three or four times daily.
See package insert.
Keep this and all drugs out of the reach
of children.
**Store below 30°C (86°F). Protect from
freezing and light.**

Exp date and lot

2220G102

Child's weight and age: 16 kg, 2 years old.

Pediatric dose: 5 mg/kg/day.

How many ml would you give?

ANSWERS

Orals

1. 4 tablets
2. ½ tablet
3. 8 ml
4. 10 ml
5. 3 tablets
6. 1 tablet
7. 225 ml of Ensure and 75 ml of water

Injectables

8. ½ ml
9. 1 ml
10. 1.25 ml
11. meperidine 0.8 ml
    atropine 1 ml
    a. Expel 0.2 ml of meperidine.
    b. Draw 1 ml of air and insert into atropine.
    c. Withdraw 1 ml of atropine.
12. 0.25 ml; tuberculin syringe
13. 1.75 ml or 1.8 ml
14. 4.6 ml of diluent (label)
    1 ml

Intravenous

15. 20–21 gtts/minute

16. 62–63 gtts/minute

17. cefamandole 6.3 ml of drug solution (mixed with 10 ml)

162 gtts/min (add the drug solution amount, 6 ml, to 75 ml)

18. cefazolin 1.5 ml

Set volumetric pump rate at 152 ml/hr. (150 ml/hr if you did not add the drug volume solution to the 75 ml.) Both answers would be correct.

19. Aq. penicillin U 300,000 = 1.9 ml

180 gtts/minute

Pediatrics

20. 10 ml

21. 3.75 ml or 4 ml

22. 1 ml

23. 5 ml

24. 18.75 ml or 19 ml

25. 10 ml

Appendices

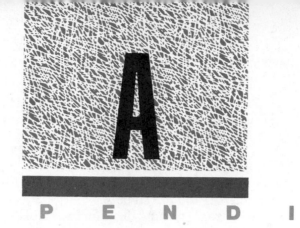

Temperature Conversion: Celsius and Fahrenheit

Two scales used to measure temperature are Fahrenheit (F) and Celsius (C), also called centigrade. Both temperature scales have boiling points and freezing points. The boiling point of Fahrenheit is 212° and the freezing point is 32°, a range of 180 (212 − 32). The boiling point of Celsius is 100° and the freezing point is 0°, a range of 100 (100 − 0). The difference of Fahrenheit to Celsius is 180 to 100 or ⁹/₅, and of Celsius to Fahrenheit is 100 to 180 or ⁵/₉.

Celsius is becoming the primary temperature scale for clinical use, so it may be necessary to convert Fahrenheit to Celsius, and Celsius to Fahrenheit. Two formulas may be used in the conversion of temperatures. Refer to the formulas as needed.

Formula A: To convert Celsius to Fahrenheit

$$F = \tfrac{9}{5}\,C + 32$$

EXAMPLE

$$35°C \text{ to Fahrenheit}$$

$$F = \tfrac{9}{5}\,C + 32$$

$$F = \tfrac{9}{5} \times 35 + 32$$

$$F = \frac{9 \times 35}{5} + 32 = \frac{315}{5} + 32$$

$$F = 63 + 32$$

$$F = 95°$$

Formula B: To convert Fahrenheit to Celsius

$$C = \tfrac{5}{9}\,(F - 32)$$

EXAMPLE

$$99°F \text{ to Celsius}$$

$$C = \tfrac{5}{9}\,(F - 32)$$

$$C = \frac{5 \times (99 - 32)}{9}$$

$$C = \frac{5 \times 67}{9} = \frac{335}{9}$$

$$C = 37.2°$$

B

Metric and Apothecary Conversion Table

Metric and Apothecary Conversions

Metric		Apothecary
Grams (g)	Milligrams (mg)	Grains (gr)
1	1000	15
0.5	500	7 ½
0.3	300 (325)	5
0.1	100	1 ½
0.06	60 (64)	1
0.03	30 (32)	½
0.02	20	⅓
0.015	15	¼
0.010	10	⅙
0.008	8	⅛
0.001	1	1/60
0.0006	0.6	1/100
0.0004	0.4	1/150
0.0003	0.3	1/200

Liquid (approximate)

30 ml (cc) = 1 fl oz (ℨ) = 2 tbsp (T) = 6–8 tsp (t) = 6–8 fl dr
15 ml (cc) = ½ fl oz   = 1 T   = 6–8 t   = 6–8 fl dr
1000 ml (cc) = 1 quart (qt) = 1 liter (L)
500 ml (cc) = 1 pint (pt)
4 ml (cc) = 1 fl dram (ℨ) = 1 tsp (t)
5 ml (cc) = 1 tsp (household)
1 ml (cc) = 15 minims = 15 drops (gtts)

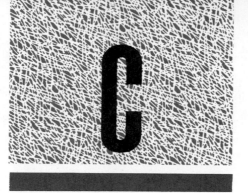

C

A P P E N D I X

Abbreviations

Abbreviations	Latin	English Meaning
aa	ana	of
a.c. (ac)	ante cibus	before meals
Ad (ad)	ad	to, up to
Aq	aqua	water
Bid (bid)	bis in die	twice a day
c̄	cum	with
cc		cubic centimeter
Caps		capsule
dr (ʒ)	drachma	dram
E.C.		enteric coated
El		elixir
Ext	extractum	extract
fl	fluidus	fluid
Gm, G, g	gramma	gram
gr	granum	grain
gtt	gutta	drop
hs	hora somni	hour of sleep
IM		intramuscular
IV		intravenous
kg	kilogram	kilogram
m	minimus	minim
mcg (μg)		microgram
mEq		milliequivalent
mg (mgm)		milligram
ml		milliliter
NPO		nothing by mouth
OD (od)	oculus dexter	right eye
o.n. or qn	omni nocte	every night
OS (os)	oculus sinister	left eye
OU (ou)	oculus uterque	each eye
oz (ʒ)		ounce
p.c. (pc)	post cibum	after meals
PO (p.o.)		by mouth
PRN	pro re nata	whenever necessary
qd	quaque die	every day
qh, Omn hor	omni hora	every hour
q1, 2, 3, 4, 6, 8h	quaque una hora	every 1, 2, 3, 4, 6, 8 hours
Qid (qid)	quarter in die	four times a day
s̄	sine	without
SC (subc, sq)		subcutaneous
Sol	solutio	solution
sos	si opus sit	once if necessary
ss	semiss	a half
Stat	statim	at once, immediate
Tab	tabella	tablet
tbsp (T)		tablespoon
Tid (tid)	ter in die	three times a day
Tr (tr)		tincture
Tsp (t)		teaspoon
ung	unguentum	ointment

Guidelines for Administration of Medications

GENERAL DRUG ADMINISTRATION

1. Check medications order with doctor's orders, Kardex, medicine card (if available), and/or other methods.

2. Check label of drug container three times.

3. Identify the patient by identification bracelet and asking patient his/her name.

4. Stay with the patient until the medication is taken.

5. Give medications last to patients who need more assistance.

6. Report drug error immediately to the head nurse and physician. Incident report is necessary.

7. Record drug given, including the name of the drug, dosage, date, time, and your initials.

8. Record drugs soon after they are given, especially stat medications. Also indicate on the drug sheet if the drug was not given.

9. Record oral intake of the amount of fluid taken with medication if the patient is on I & O.

10. Be aware that nurses have a right to question drug orders. Physicians are responsible for medication order, dosage, and route for drug administration. Nurses are responsible for administered medications.

11. Administer drug within 30 minutes of its prescribed time (30 minutes before prescribed time or 30 minutes after).

12. Do not guess when preparing medication. Check order sheet if drug order is not clear. Call the pharmacist, physician, and/or nursing supervisor if in doubt.

13. Do not give drugs poured by others.

14. Do not leave drug tray or cart out of sight.

15. Know that patients have a right to refuse medication. If possible, ascertain why the patient refuses the medication. Report refusal to take medications.

16. Check if patient states that he/she has an allergy to the drug or a drug group.

17. Know the seven *Rights:* right drug, right dose, right route, right time, right patient, right of patient to know reason for drug, and right of patient to refuse medication.

ORAL MEDICATIONS

1. Wash hands before preparing oral medications.

2. Pour tablet or capsule into drug container's cap (top) and NOT into

the hand. Drugs prepared for unit dose can be opened at the time of administration in the patient's room. Discard drugs that are dropped on the floor.

3. Pour liquids on a flat surface at eye level with thumbnail on medicine cup line.

4. Do not mix liquids with tablets or liquids with liquids in the same container. Tablets and capsules may be put in the same container *except* for oral narcotics, digoxin, PRN, and stat medications.

5. Do not pour drugs from labels that are difficult to read.

6. Do not return poured medication to its container. Properly discard poured medication if not used.

7. Do not transfer medication from one container to another.

8. Pour liquid medications from the side opposite the bottle's label to avoid spilling medicine on the label.

9. Dilute liquid medications that irritate gastric mucosa, e.g., potassium products, or that could discolor/damage tooth enamel, e.g., SSKI, or have patient take the drug with meals.

10. Offer ice chips prior to distasteful medications to numb the taste buds.

11. Assist patient into upright position when administering oral medications. Stay with patient until medication is taken.

12. Give at least 50 to 100 ml of oral fluids with medications unless the patient has a fluid restriction. It helps to ensure that medication reaches the stomach.

INJECTABLE MEDICATIONS

1. Wash hands before preparing injectable medications.

2. Select the proper syringe and needle size for the type of medication to be administered.

3. Select the injection site according to the drug.

4. Check for drug compatibility before mixing drugs in the same syringe.

5. Check expiration date before preparing medication. If in doubt, check with the pharmacist.

6. Check label on drug container to determine method(s) for drug administration, i.e., IM, IV, SC.

7. Do not give parenteral medications that are cloudy, are discolored, or have precipitated.

8. Aspirate plunger before injecting medication. If blood returns, STOP, withdraw needle, and prepare new solution. Check the policy of your institution.

9. Do not massage injection site if using Z-track method, intradermal, heparin, or any anticoagulant solution.

10. Do not administer injections in inflamed and edematous tissues or to lesion (moles, birthmarks, scar) sites.

11. Recognize that individuals experiencing edema, shock, or poor circulation will have a very slow tissue absorption rate following intramuscular injection.

12. Discard liquid drugs into the sink or toilet, NOT into the trash can.

13. Discard needles safely into the proper container.

14. Refrigerate unused reconstituted powdered medication in vials.

15. Discard unused solution in ampules. Ampules once opened cannot be reused.

16. Do not administer IM medications subcutaneously. Sloughing of the subcutaneous tissue could occur.

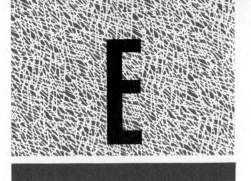

Nomograms

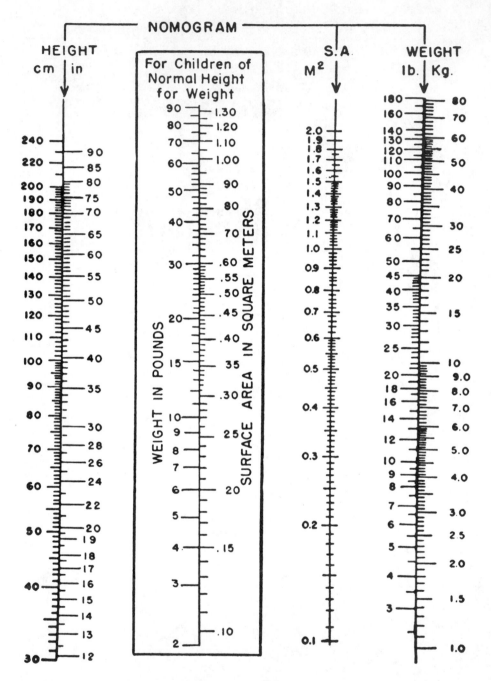

West Nomogram: For Infants and Children.

Directions: (1) Find height. (2) Find weight. (3) Draw a straight line connecting the height and weight, and where the line intersects on the SA column is the body surface area (m²).

(From Behrman, R.E., and Vaughan, V.C.: Nelson Textbook of Pediatrics, Philadelphia, W.B. Saunders Co., 1987.)

BODY SURFACE AREA OF CHILDREN

Nomogram for determination of body surface area from height and weight

Height	Body surface area (BSA)	Weight

Directions: (1) Find height in height column on left. (2) Find weight in weight column on right. (3) Draw a straight line connecting the height and weight. Where the line intersects on the BSA column is the body surface area (m²).

(From Lentner, C. (ed.): Geigy Scientific Tables, 8th ed., Basle, Switzerland, Ciba-Geigy, 1981, pp. 226-227.)

BODY SURFACE AREA OF ADULTS

Nomogram for determination of body surface area from height and weight

Height	Body surface area (BSA)	Weight

The nomogram consists of three vertical scales:

Height

cm | inch

200 — 79 in
78
195 — 77
76
190 — 75
74
185 — 73
72
180 — 71
70
175 — 69
68
170 — 67
66
165 — 65
64
160 — 63
62
155 — 61
60
150 — 59
58
145 — 57
56
140 — 55
54
135 — 53
52
130 — 51
50
125 — 49
48
120 — 47
46
115 — 45
44
110 — 43
42
105 — 41
40
cm 100 — 39 in

Body surface area (BSA) — m^2

2.80
2.70
2.60
2.50
2.40
2.30
2.20
2.10
2.00
1.95
1.90
1.85
1.80
1.75
1.70
1.65
1.60
1.55
1.50
1.45
1.40
1.35
1.30
1.25
1.20
1.15
1.10
1.05
1.00
0.95
0.90
0.86 m^2

Weight

kg | lb

150 — 330
145 — 320
140 — 310
135 — 300
130 — 290
125 — 280
120 — 270
115 — 260
110 — 250
105 — 240
100 — 230
95 — 220
90 — 210
85 — 200
80 — 190
75 — 180
70 — 170
65 — 160
60 — 150
55 — 140
50 — 130
45 — 120
40 — 110
35 — 105
100
95
90
85
80
75
70
kg 30 — 66 lb

Directions: (1) Find height in height column on left. (2) Find weight in weight column on right. (3) Draw a straight line connecting the height and weight. Where the line intersects on the BSA column is the body surface area (m^2).

(From Lentner, C. (ed.): Geigy Scientific Tables, 8th ed., Basle, Switzerland, Ciba-Geigy, 1981, pp. 226–227.)

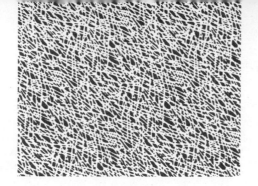

Index

Note: Page numbers in *italics* refer to illustrations. Page numbers followed by (t) refer to tables.